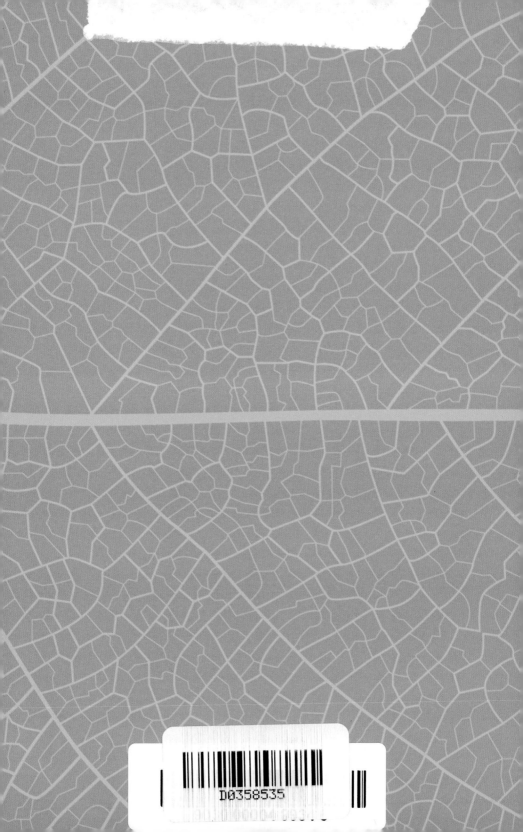

THE
TREE
CLIMBER'S
GUIDE

THE
TREE
CLIMBER'S
GUIDE

ADVENTURES IN THE URBAN CANOPY

JACK COOKE

Illustrated by Jennifer Pitchers

HarperCollins*Publishers*

HarperCollins*Publishers*
1 London Bridge Street
London SE1 9GF

www.harpercollins.co.uk

First published by HarperCol

10 9 8 7 6 5 4 3 2 1

Text © Jack Cooke 2016
Illustrations © Jennifer Pitchers 2016

Jack Cooke asserts the moral right to be
identified as the author of this work

A catalogue record of this book is
available from the British Library

HB ISBN 978-0-00-815391-5

Printed and bound in Great Britain by
Clays Ltd, St Ives plc

The activities discussed in this book can be very dangerous.
Any person should approach these activities with caution
and appropriate supervision.

MIX
Paper from
responsible sources
FSC
www.fsc.org   **FSC C007454**

FSC™ is a non-profit international organisation established to promote
the responsible management of the world's forests. Products carrying the
FSC label are independently certified to assure consumers that they come
from forests that are managed to meet the social, economic and
ecological needs of present and future generations, and other
controlled sources.

Find out more about HarperCollins and the environment at
www.harpercollins.co.uk/green

To my mother, who has a great love of trees
and a mortal fear of heights

'Back to the trees!' shouted Uncle Vanya.
'Back to nature!'

The Evolution Man, Or,
How I Ate My Father, Roy Lewis

Contents

65   City Parks

187 Streets, Roundabouts & Rooftops

203 Seasons

211 Open Ground

THE
TREE
CLIMBER'S
GUIDE

Introduction

One thing we rarely do in the city is look up. Only time and weather seem to invade our thoughts as we tramp the urban mile. We may raise our eyes to coming rain or the hours called by clocks, but little else breaks our focus on the way to and from – our eternal quest for convenience.

There is another dimension to the city, a world far removed but close at hand. It is a place of limitless space and light, and a simple antidote to the crowds. When we escape into this realm our senses are replenished; we taste cleaner air and see further than the end of the road. Where does this unlikely utopia lie? All around and above you, in the lofty, green canopy of the city's trees.

The city I inhabit is not so very different from any other. Like all cities it is sculpted from the same fixed matter: steel and glass, stone and brick. But like all cities it is underpinned and overhung by nature. Everything man-made is dug into the soil, and beneath the street a vast network of roots threads the land.

I have climbed trees in London, but wherever you live you cannot be far from a low branch. The location of a tree is not as important as the act of climbing; you could be scaling a pine in Glasgow or an oak in Rome. Trees offer a way up and out of every city in which they thrive.

There are an estimated seven million trees growing across London, almost a tree for every man, woman and child living in the city. They are as varied and individual as London's human inhabitants, from hoary old veterans to assertive young saplings, and as a would-be climber of their branches you have a lot of introductions to make.

The premium commodity in cities is space – space and the terrible lack of it. A recurring bass line in our media is the ever-increasing rent to be paid for one house, one flat, one room, one box. London's human-built habitation has become inflated beyond recognition, yet the city retains a set of residents who enjoy its most exclusive addresses, the best access and architecture, and the finest views. These lucky few are not the skyscraper elite in their capsules of glass and steel, nor the sprawling mansion dwellers of Hampstead and Chelsea. There exists another kind of penthouse, and its occupants – the humble bird and beast – live in it for free.

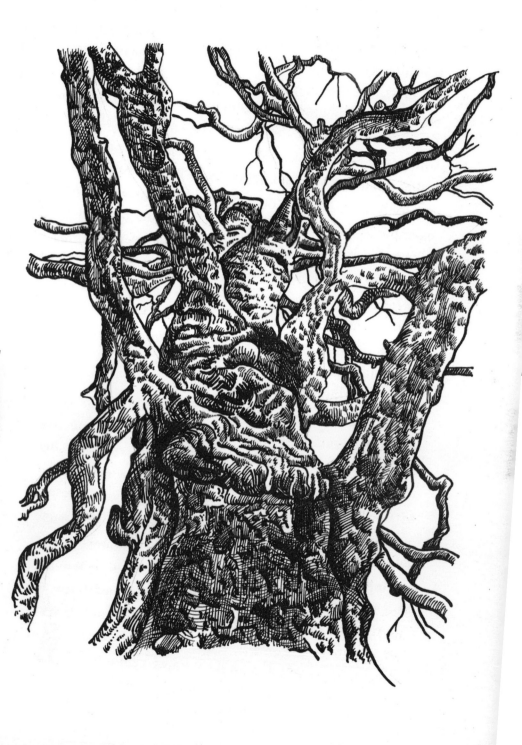

They are rooted in the city but apart from it; the space is in the tree tops.

London is a verdant metropolis, with more parks and green spaces than any other capital of comparable size. At whatever compass point of the city you find yourself, you're never far from a break in the asphalt and a climbable tree. Climb a few feet up and out, and you're suddenly suspended above the crowds, alone on your perch and enjoying a fresh breeze.

This book aims to give the reader a new A–Z, one that runs from Ash to Zelkova, offering escape wherever you find yourself. It is not a survey but a personal selection, representing the very tip of a deep arboreal iceberg. Variety is at the heart of climbing trees, and I hope to inspire others to go out and find their own citadels.

There are, of course, obstacles to us claiming the city's forgotten paradise but, fortunately, they exist largely in our own heads. The two greatest of these, fear and shame, hinder and guard us at all times. Taken together they form a powerful anchor that keeps most of us firmly grounded.

The first emotion is natural and healthy. Fear is the backbone of survival and no bad thing. It seems rational to look up into a fifty-foot oak, the wind shaking its crown, and decide that you are better placed on terra firma. But if we analyse this fear, we see that it can also be limiting; it's a feeling based more on a phobia of the unknown than a fear of falling. Although we no longer possess the mighty forearms of our hominid ancestors, human biology still makes us remarkably adept tree climbers. We came from the trees and we can return to them. Starting small, you'll find that oak, ash, pine and cedar offer ladder-like ascents on firm boughs. Your balance and agility might be better than you suspect.

As we get older and grow out of many childhood fears, we develop others. We no longer dread what lies beneath the bed, but those who once sprung off trampolines now fear anything higher than a stepladder. Mounting the kitchen sideboard or reaching to close a window we find ourselves suddenly dizzy, reeling at a sheer drop of three feet. In such instances vertigo is an irrational response. Just like the rabbit in the headlights, it serves no evolutionary purpose; fear is there to be subordinated to our willpower. The humanzee may overcometh.

The second obstacle, shame, is the harder to surmount. This is because it's so deeply ingrained, a tragic part of our social conditioning. There seems to be a common perception that climbing trees is not at all respectable. Like so many precepts that bind us as adults, it's 'just not what grown-ups do'. Long labelled the preserve of children by the unimaginative, an adult in a tree is drunk, deranged, suicidal – or a combination of all three. We are denied the pleasures of the trees by our own self-policing, by the roles we assume in this protective and circumscribing society.

For a grown man or woman, then, climbing a tree is out of the question. No matter how much he or she recounts green-at-the-knee tales of childhood climbs, no responsible citizen would shimmy up a willow. On the rare occasions adults do venture into the trees it's usually to impress friends and show off, which should never be the inspiration or goal of climbing.

Conquering fear and shame is as much about rediscovering our beginnings as abandoning our tame maturity. The adult measures enjoyment against the future, pausing at the foot of the tree, while the child lives in the moment. The instant that you value a new set of clothes over a new experience you have forgotten how to enjoy yourself. We must grow as children, not shrink as adults.

If you are ready to master these emotions, a new haven lies waiting for you. Before long you can be ten, thirty or fifty feet above your surroundings. It is an addictive experience, and the best trees can be enjoyed from their lowest branch to their topmost. Swing out onto a low perch and dangle your legs a few feet off the ground. Climb a little higher and edge out of sight. Still higher, and you will find different windows opening on the world below, a new perspective on the city with every branch you grasp.

Many are the poets who have stood in the shade of a great tree and proclaimed its beauty, but what they behold is a mere fraction of the whole. By climbing, we engage all our senses. The textures of different barks and the suppleness of branches that bend under our weight are a stark contrast to the synthetic nature of the world we inhabit at ground level. Pausing in a tree top we can tune in to an alternative soundscape, a world of subtle variation unnoticed in the cacophony of the street; the heavy sigh of a branch buffeted by a lorry's slipstream or a full head of leaves catching the wind off the river.

Only once, in all the trees I've climbed across the city, have I found someone sitting in the top of one. The man I encountered was small, grey and smiling. He was at least sixty, dressed in suit trousers with his shirt untucked and a jacket and tie hanging on the branch below him. Once we had gotten over our mutual surprise – and I'd taken a subordinate perch – we began talking. This man was no great libertarian, no anarchist or antichrist. He was simply a lawyer on a lunch break having his sandwich in an ash tree. This decision, to eat at altitude above the packed square of the park, was not a radical one. To me this man was following the most natural inclination in the world – a desire for breathing space and a different point of view.

London was built on a swamp, and it doesn't take much height to achieve a good vantage point. But there are trees in the capital where, with little skill or strength but due care, the committed explorer can climb high above their surroundings. There is perhaps no feeling quite like sticking your head through the topmost branches of a tree, pushing through a pine canopy or reaching for the last bunch of oak leaves. You emerge from a dense network of branches below to an open sky and boundless views stretching away on every side. Beneath, filtered through summer green or the bare branches of winter, are the passing crowns of people's heads: blonde, brunette, bald. The ground is flat and clean, and the world about is round.

It is these living lookouts – and the thousands of new views of the city they provide, open and free to all – that are at the heart of this book. Office blocks shimmer through the fronds of a cedar, skyscrapers loom above a green crown and the long lines of tenements dwindle into the distance.

Trees deliver us from the banal, and reaching the top of one is like coming up for air and breaking the bubble of our timetabled lives. Their physical complexity, together with the courage needed to climb them, liberates thought and offers a wealth of natural knowledge. The treeline acts as a defence against the darker parts of urban living and the canopy is an inviolate place, a still room for reflection amid the constant rush of city life.

There is nothing better for seeing the world more clearly than removing yourself a little distance from it. So the next time the city overwhelms you, when you feel hemmed in or shut out, remember to look up. Escape is at hand, reprieve is at foot; you are never far from ascension.

The Inner Gibbon

A Short History of Climbing Trees

A house in which rain does not fall, a place in which
spears are not feared, as open as if in a garden without
a fence around it.

The Ivied Tree-top, unknown Irish author,
9th century AD

Not so very long ago you and I were both exceptional climbers. We breezed through the trees, living, hunting and sleeping in the greenery. Bridging the gap between branches was
second nature to our ancestors, and they wouldn't have

thought twice about jumping the void to secure a good breakfast. The tree tops were their temple and tabernacle.

This continued for many tens of millions of happy years. Then, one fateful afternoon, we stepped down from the heights and began our life as ground dwellers. Soon to become the baldest of the apes, we abandoned the very thing that had sustained us for countless generations, deciding instead to seek our future on two feet.

Whatever forced this great transition, climate or curiosity, the outcome has clearly been a terrible mistake. We traded brawn for brains, opposable toes for stilettos, and sacrificed instinct and sustainable habitat for an intelligence that would culminate, roughly thirteen million years later, in the ability to doubt ourselves.

Even after making the era-defining choice of no longer living in the trees, our ancestors most likely returned to them in times of need. Where else would you flee when being chased across the African savannah by the larger of the ground-dwelling predators? Indeed you might only be reading this due to the climbing skill-set of your very great-grandmother, which enabled her to escape the jaws of various ravenous beasts (or at least those unable to give chase up trees).

But there came a time when we no longer needed to ascend to survive. The invention of fire, tools and, more recently, television has made climbing trees largely surplus to human requirements. Although a number of diligent tribes continued to seek food and shelter in the canopy, living exclusively up high became a rare lifestyle choice; those still clinging to the branches in the 21st century are few and far between. Our relationship with the trees has changed from one of co-existence to increasing exploitation.

In spite of our great descent, the lure of climbing trees has persisted. Throughout history, thinkers and dreamers have returned to the forest compelled by a shared ancestral memory. Trees bring out a powerful homing instinct in many of us and we gravitate towards them, a part of us, perhaps, longing to return to our former existence. The poetic image of the dying soldier comes to mind, dragging himself to the base of a tree before expelling a final breath. Trees remain linked to our concept of a life cycle, their death and rebirth analogous to humankind's own measurement of time. The Green Man of pre-Christian symbolism, a kind of arboreal divinity, is an enduring mark of this tie to the trees. Living faces and hollow skulls sprout leaves from mouth and ears, a relic of our former union with the vegetable world.

If we search for tree dwellers down the millennia we find curious instances of men and women climbing back into the canopy. Consider the druids, most venerated of ancient Britons and the policy makers of their day. If we credit Pliny's *Natural History*, one of their sacred rituals was running up an oak tree under a full moon to cut down fistfuls of mistletoe. Only the druids were permitted to climb the hallowed trees, a sure sign of the ancients' veneration for this noble art.

In AD 436, a slightly awkward teenager called Simeon decided to climb a pillar and spend the rest of his life sitting on top of it. Although historians have immortalised him as a man seeking spiritual enlightenment, I think Simeon was following a nagging instinct to nest. Hounded by other lost souls seeking spiritual advice, he chose to escape the world by climbing above it.

Simeon's life up high inspired a cult of pillar-squatting Christians known as *stylites*, 'pillar dwellers'; others took to the trees, hiding away from the world in hollow trunks or climbing branches to nest like birds in the tree tops. Early icons display barefoot monks perched happily in the canopy, with various followers bringing them food and drink. These men became known as *dendrites*, 'people of the tree', and most famous among them was David, more formally known as Saint David of Thessalonika. He spent three years living in an almond tree, nominally talking to God but also enjoying the nuts and the view. Spend long enough in the branches and you too may find yourself beatified.

Scaling trees was certainly still commonplace in the Middle Ages. *The Fates of Men*, an Old English poem of the 8th century, provides a fascinating list of fatal misfortunes that might befall your average Anglo-Saxon. Most of these we can readily accept as unremarkable for the age: being devoured by a wolf, being pierced by a spear, dying through storm, starvation or war. Some of the documented fates even have modern-day parallels, like the man 'maddened with mead' who dies in the Dark Ages' equivalent of a bar brawl.

In among all this misery is death by falling from a tree. It seems an odd fate to include in a list of everyday dangers:

One from the top of a tree in the woods
Without feathers shall fall, but he flies none the less,
Swoops in descent till he seems no longer
The forest tree's fruit; at its foot on the ground
He sinks in silence, his soul departed –
On the roots now lies his lifeless body.

The bard's lyrical account of a fatal slip implies that a number of people could still be found hanging around in the tree tops. In those heady days several different vocations might have lured our forebears back into the canopy: drovers would climb up beech and ash, collecting leaves as forage for their cattle, and medieval falconers seem to have spent half their lives chasing wayward hawks off high branches. Plucky soldiers would also have scaled the heights to get the lie of the land. Before the advent of balloons or drones, climbing a tree was as good a way as any of spying on your neighbour.

Fast forward a thousand years and some truly remarkable tree climbers emerge from the 18th century. In the forests of France and Germany hunting parties discovered several instances of children living wild, subsisting alone deep in the woods. Peter the Wild Boy, who later became a court celebrity in England, was discovered 'walking on his hands and feet, climbing trees like a squirrel, and feeding on grass and moss'. Attempts to capture him resulted in the 'savage' taking refuge in a tree that had to be cut down in order to catch him. A similar story emerged in the 1790s, when three hunters came across a boy covered in scars living in the woods near Saint-Sernin-sur-Rance. Again, when they attempted to capture him the child's first instinct was to climb a tree, from which he was subsequently dragged down. Both Peter and Victor, the second boy, were found to be living on forest flora – bark, berries and roots – and seemed to have reverted to nesting in the trees.

During the course of their subsequent lives, unhappily paraded as oddities, they often attempted to escape back into the forest. Although their legendary stories have a tragic origin as they were most likely abandoned, both boys demonstrate the remarkable ability of humans to survive in the wild and our instinctual preference for seeking shelter in the trees.

More extraordinary than either case is that of Marie-Angélique Memmie Le Blanc. In 1731, on the outskirts of the French commune of Songy, a thief clothed in animal skins was found stealing apples from an orchard. The villagers set a bulldog upon the intruder, who was said to have struck it dead with a single blow. Pursued by a mob, the mysterious figure vanished back into the nearby forest, swinging from branch to branch across the tree tops. A vengeful party was soon sent after the thief, who turned out to be a girl of nineteen living off raw meat and fish, and sleeping in the canopy of a tree.

'The Shepherd's Beast', as the new marvel was known, spent the following years of her life sequestered in a series of convents. This sudden change to a cloistered living space and cooked food destroyed her previously robust constitution. Within a few weeks all of her teeth fell out and she was given

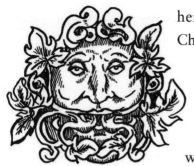 her new name, redolent of Christian morality.

Unique among such cases, Marie-Angélique recovered the power of speech and was 'integrated' back into society, where her full story slowly came to light. She was found to be of Native American origin and had been living wild for a decade or more. Her return was considered a triumph of civilisation, and her restoration to speech a victory for rational thought. In reality, her captors had undone years of instinctual living, caging the most well-adapted tree dweller since the age of the Great Ape.

In the 20th century the number of children and adults climbing trees appears to have been declining down the generations. We already seem divorced from our grandparents, to whom exploring was an essential part of play. David Haffner, a climber from Coventry in his mid-seventies, sent me an account of his childhood escapades on the city's outskirts. In this glorious 1950s tale of derring-do, a boy named Tom climbs a tall elm to reach a linnet's nest high up in its branches. Thirty feet above the ground, egged on by his companions, Tom makes a desperate move, slips from a branch and comes crashing down into a thicket of elm saplings. Miraculously, he survives with no more than a few cuts and bruises. David's story is one of many from an era when a 'boys-will-be-boys' mentality prevailed. For all its potential horror, the tale is a love letter to natural adventure and the antithesis of today's risk-averse culture.

Another example of the generation gap is found in a curious American legal case brought to court in 1919. The lawsuit involved a power company forced to pay damages to the father of a boy killed while climbing a tree on common ground, through which electricity cables had been strung. The judgment concluded that the boy had broken no laws and that 'courts further realise that children are apt to climb trees'. It's hard to imagine a similar case today, when children and adults alike are more liable to be plugged into headphones and screens than found up in the branches. A child scaling an oak adjoining power lines would now be served with an ASBO, that is if the same tree had not long ago been removed. There are currently several laws against climbing trees in public spaces, and as recently as 2012 Enfield council attempted to ban the practice altogether in its parks and green spaces.

In spite of these societal shifts, it is hardly surprising that the impulse to climb trees remains strong; the art is lost but the memory lives on. Abandon a small child in the depths of a forest and, after much sobbing at their predicament, you might well find them up a tree. Walk through a city park on a summer's day and observe groups of toddlers crowded around the base of tall oaks, desperately trying to reach the branches. Their parents, each some distance apart, will probably be playing on their phones. We are less cut off from our deep history than from our own childhood.

How then do we stop ourselves devolving from climbing children to earthbound adults? Happily, the damage done is only superficial and it is easier to discard the short years of our nurture than the fundamental draw of our nature. Climbing, we regress back beyond our industrial present, rejoining the scramblers of the past and retracing our ancestral tree into its shrouded pre-history. The hard surfaces of the city's streets yield to an older kingdom, where tunnels of webbed branch and briar superimpose themselves on the human-built environment. Tomorrow, you can step out of your front door and into a tree, reclaiming a forgotten birthright; it only takes a moment to return over the threshold of the first branch.

My own journey back to the trees began on a day shadowed by storm cloud, the end of summer with a fierce wind funnelling through central London and sweeping all before it. I was working in an office housed on the top floor of an old terrace. The building faced Regent's Park but a brick parapet blocked the window view, built to hide the old servant's quarters from the high society of the day. Although we could glimpse a slice of sky, the park remained invisible. Our only other reminder of the world outside was a London plane that grew to the full height of the building, the tips of its highest branches scratching at the window panes.

That morning the weather had caused chaos in the artificial order of our office. Torrential rain had opened a hidden sluice gate in the building's plasterwork and a river of water descended, channelled by the carpet between the desks into a great indoor delta. The building's caretaker had bravely opened a skylight in search of the flood's source but returned unenlightened. Foolishly, he left the ladder and the key to the roof behind him. When the office emptied out at lunch I seized my chance to finally see the view.

Stepping out onto the lead roof, I was nearly blown clean over the edge by the wind. I latched on to the skylight's surround like a limpet and gazed in awe at the panorama beyond the gutter. Regent's Park stretched across my entire field of vision, the summer canopy conjoined into a single roiling green sea, the tree tops looking like another world hanging over London. Everywhere, thick foliage performed a furious dance, the willow's long locks thrashing against the oak's Afro, the whole scene bursting with a life far removed from my own. In contrast, my desk was locked in a desensitised world, a static realm where the only movements were the twitching of plastic mice. It was a rare awakening.

In one of life's happy coincidences I had recently begun reading the adventures of Cosimo, a little-known hero sprung from the imagination of Italo Calvino. In his 1957 novel *The Baron in the Trees*, the author describes a mythical Italian valley where the forest grows so thick that each tree interlaces with the next. Into this wooded wonderland the figure of Cosimo is released, a kind of 18th-century Tarzan. Climbing out of his father's dining-room window in protest at being forced to eat snails, Cosimo disappears into the canopy and refuses to return. His regular aerial pastimes include reading and hunting, then later, seducing women and starting revolutions. He lives out the rest of his days far from the circumscribed routine of his former life. Over the course of the novel he acquires 'bandy legs and long monkey-like arms', returning to the physiognomy of his ape ancestors while cultivating a tree-top philosophy all of his own. He never again sets foot on the ground, not even in death.

Under the thick summer verdure of Regent's Park, Cosimo's 'Republic of Arborea', a land where roaming the canopy was as easy as crossing the street, did not seem so distant. I imagined opening the office window, five floors off the ground, climbing over the parapet and leaping onto the outstretched arm of the plane tree. By a series of bridges and ladders I'd make my way down and out across the street, dropping from the final branch into the elusive Eden on the far side. In reality I took the lift.

Five minutes later I found myself walking across the wind-swept park lawns. Here and there the branches of separate trees linked overhead, and I pictured Cosimo skipping across the divides. Although careful planting schemes displaced the natural wilderness in my head, the violent weather made rose beds and box hedges look as wild as an untamed wood. Before long the rain returned and I ran for the shelter of a pine.

Under the canopy the sound of the storm intensified, a waterfall now ringing the tree's perimeter. Placing a hand on the lowest branch level with my chest, I looked up into the pine's conical interior. Stretching far above, the crown seemed like a safe haven even as its uppermost branches swayed out of sight. Cautiously, I stepped over the first rung and out onto the next, the tree's thick arms offering a fixed ladder. My confidence soon began to grow, and before long I was high above the park and sitting on a wide cross-bar. Looking down on a blustery London from this new habitat, I felt strangely protected. To the south, the city rolled out beyond the borders of the park and, although less than ten minutes' walk from my office, I already felt a world apart.

Returning to work, sodden and with sap-covered hands, I struggled to settle back into my daily routine. The material pleasures of city life paled in comparison with my experience of climbing the tree. Sitting in the storm-tossed pine, my whole body cradled by the branches, had awoken a dormant escapist. The four walls of my office were no longer protection against the weather but an insentient cage. Weeks later I was still dwelling on that same five minutes spent perched in the tree, and every lunch break I strayed back into the park, searching for a new tower to climb. These brief interludes between hours of phone calls, emails and spreadsheets became more protracted, and my colleagues' suspicions deepened. I would return to work with a head full of curling branches and feathered skylines, and when there was no alternative but to sit at my desk I searched online for traces of other climbers in the city. But I found none. The only men and women who seemed to scale the trees were, like Cosimo, the figments of others' imaginations.

The history of climbing trees is composed as much from myth as recorded deed. Our memories of an older, entangled world, a life lived in the forests, express themselves across the full scope of our fiction and fairy tale.

Alongside Cosimo are other heroes who cast aside the everyday and returned to the trees. Memorable among these are Robin, John and Harold in the wildwood classic *Brendon Chase*, a band of brothers who escape the guardianship of their 'iron-grey' aunt and disappear into the woods for eight months, refusing to return to school. Hiding out in the hollowed trunk of an old oak, the three boys are enriched by their experience of living wild; making beds of bracken, swimming in hollows, stealing wild honey and climbing trees. The novel contrasts the daily wonder of the woods with the strictures of the 'civilised' world. In one of its most vivid scenes, Robin climbs a giant pine in order to steal an egg from a honey buzzard's nest. The terror he feels in the topmost branches, hanging high above the other trees, is contrasted with the solace of the thick trunk and its rough bark. In both *The Baron in the Trees* and *Brendon Chase*, climbing trees is a way of resisting the constraints of society, whether these are the stifling influence of a controlling father or the numbing routine of a 1920s boarding school.

Many of our popular legends spring from the forest, the dwelling place of elves and witches, dryads and nymphs, and a whole cast of characters born of folktale, from *Baba Yaga* to *Little Red Riding Hood*. In this rich tradition, climbing trees often serves as a refuge from the evils of the world.

One of my favourites climbing tales is *The Minpins*, the last story Roald Dahl wrote before his death. The protagonist, Little Billy, ignores his mother's words of warning and is tempted into the ominous Forest of Sin, a brooding presence on the far side of the village lane. Lost in the trees, he finds himself pursued by a terrifying monster of the forest floor, the notorious 'Bloodsucking, Toothplucking, Stonechucking Spittler'. In desperation, Billy jumps into the only tree offering salvation and, terrified, climbs branch over branch, higher and higher, only stopping when he is completely exhausted. Looking around him, Billy discovers the emerald interior of what looks, in my old illustrated edition, like a giant beech. He watches in fascination as hundreds of little doors open in the bark of the branches, windows into the interior of a miniature city, the realm of the Minpins. Befriending this diminutive race, Billy discovers a self-sufficient society at one with nature. The Minpins even harness the flight of birds to transport them from tree to tree, and our hero leaves the beech on the back of an improbably massive swan, soaring over the dreaded Spittler and triumphantly leading the monster to its doom in the depths of a lake. The story is a wonderful enticement to children and adults alike: climb a tree and you will escape the horrors of the world, both real and imagined.

The upper branches not only contain new worlds but serve as doorways to others. In Enid Blyton's *Faraway Tree* series, every journey to the heights of this woodland giant reveals a different landscape, realms only accessible by climbing to the top and into the clouds. There are other tales of magical climbing plants and trees that appear overnight, from Jack's fabled beanstalk to the enchanted forest in Miyazaki's *My Neighbour Totoro*. These supernatural growths are a refuge from the hard reality of earthbound lives.

Some of our great science-fiction fables also have arboreal roots. In *Hothouse*, Brian Aldiss portrays a dystopian future in which vegetable life has taken over the planet and all but a handful of animal species are long since extinct. The survivors subsist in the arms of a giant banyan tree covering most of the continent, battling against a host of vegetable predators. Amid all the ecological upheaval, bands of humans have reverted to a nesting existence, living in 'nuthuts' attached to the undersides of branches. When a character dies they are elegiacally described as having 'fallen to the green'.

All these threads of storytelling are bound up in branches, and by climbing we pay homage to our heroes. Whether following Cosimo or countless others, we connect to a long and rich tradition. In cities, trees offer escape for mind and body, and we come closer to legend every time we step into them.

Today, climbing trees seems to be a theme that's fading from our literature, perhaps as adults and children in turn forsake the tree tops. Where still woven into fiction it is liable to become pure fantasy, as impossible as chasing dragon tails. Could this be the harbinger of a future in which, if we climb trees at all, it will only be among the pixels of our screens rather than under the power of our own limbs? Fear the day when we are so enraptured by our own invention that we no longer interact at all with the organic world. The instinct to climb trees may finally and irreversibly be erased.

Travelling around London, I find my grim vision alleviated by the cracks in the pavement beneath trees, where thick roots have broken concrete slabs and nature has outmuscled the man-made. Nothing gives me more joy than the sight of a water main ruptured in two or a new sports car crushed under a fallen branch. Perhaps there exists an alternative future in which the vegetable world reasserts itself in our everyday consciousness, trees becoming as prized as our castles and cathedral towers. All it takes is the tap of a branch to open our eyes to another world hanging overhead.

Green Fingers

So it is also with trees, whose nature it is to stand up high. Though thou pull any bough down to the earth, such as thou mayest bend; as soon as thou lettest it go, so soon springs it up and moves towards its kind.
Metres of Boethius (King Alfred's prose version)

This book will not tell you how to climb trees. You are, believe it or not, a natural climber, and the wherewithal to conquer nature's scaffold lies deeply ingrained in your DNA. Rewind the clock to the first tree you ever climbed; can you remember where it stood and if it stands today? Never were you more likely to fall out of a tree than when you first climbed one; the intervening years may have stiffened muscles and added gut but the way into the trees remains open.

Not long ago I found myself stuck halfway up a giant cedar. I had struggled up the bare lower trunk, wrestling with a thick covering of ivy. Arriving at the first branches and faced with the final ascent, I found my limbs frozen stiff. A friend, who had already nimbly picked his way to the summit, looked down on me through the fronds with a self-satisfied grin. I had one knee balanced on a branch, an arm wrapped around the trunk and my nose wedged in the bark. A buttock was braced against another bough and I was bleeding from a cut to my right ear.

Climbing trees is an all-body pursuit that engages every part of your anatomy; it's not unusual to find your forehead pressed hard against a thorny trunk, buttressing the rest of your body weight, or your legs locked off around a tree limb. The joy of climbing trees comes from their barely ordered chaos; branches balance each other, but every tree is its own bedlam. Getting hopelessly lost in this arboreal cobweb is the whole point.

Inevitably, upper-body strength helps. If you can do seventeen pull-ups hanging from the little finger of your left hand, then you have an advantage over the rest of us. The skill-set of a seasoned alpinist can be applied to bark but the novice is not ill-equipped. When exploring trees, the finer points of technique are subordinated to the haphazard joy of the climb.

This is a book with a strictly amateur philosophy. The closest many adults get to climbing trees in the 21st century is by paying for the privilege – even something so patently non-monetary has been ingeniously commercialised. You can be parted from your cash to be winched into the canopy, a harness tightened mercilessly around your genitals and a plastic helmet fused to your hair. With the overriding pain in your crotch, and your instructor swinging like an angry pendulum between you and the tree, there is little if any time for appreciating the scenery.

Such equipment might be useful for conquering otherwise unclimbable summits, the coast redwoods of Oregon or California, but the amateur goes into the trees as his ancestors left them. The examples in this book are for the spur of the moment, to be climbed with no other tools than your own hands and feet.

We live in a dangerous age in which some of our most natural and time-honoured pursuits have been rebranded. Swimming anywhere other than a plumbed and chlorinated pool and what you might have previously considered camping are now both given the prefix 'wild'. There is no true wilderness left in Britain, so we can assume this new perception exists to distinguish between pool and pond, campsite and moorland. More disturbingly, however, the terms imply you somehow have to be 'wild' to partake. This could not be less true of climbing trees, an undertaking for anyone with the time and inclination.

In London, gaining a branch takes perseverance. Many of the finest specimens are impossible to scale with the simple gifts that Mother Nature bestowed upon us. The city's trees have been clipped and coppiced, pruned and pollarded, shorn of their bottom branches and trimmed to a fault. London's councils and park keepers do a noble job of hairdressing, often vital to the tree's health but at a terrible cost to the aspirant climber.

How many trees I have longed to climb and left regretfully: the silver lime by London Wall, high among Roman ruins, or the soaring arms of a copper beech in Kensal Green, shadowing the cemetery. Walking through Ranelagh Gardens or London Fields, I look longingly at centuries-old trunks, bereft of a single handhold. All across the city, countless London planes elude the climber, their complex crowns arching out of reach above the roof line.

The first and greatest challenge is reaching the lowest branch of any given tree; this is the key that opens the trapdoor to the attic, and the toughest part of almost every climb is found right at the outset. In order to gain the canopy no method is too unorthodox. Grapple and grope, claw and haul your way in; I have used tooth and nail in desperate bids to ascend a coveted tree. Sheer bloody-mindedness will often prevail, and no true tree climber gives a damn about their dignity.

The greatest single aid is a tall friend, a running jump being no substitute for a reliable shoulder. Pick climbing accomplices of a sizeable stature and you'll transform your reach, elusive branches now becoming easily attainable. Elevated from my humble five foot seven to the realm of a giant by taller men, hundreds of remote tree tops have fallen within my grasp. Many of these friends have no inclination to follow me into the trees, but for every unwilling climber there's a committed pedestal.

There are, however, benefits to climbing alone. Just as the solo walker absorbs more of their immediate surroundings, so too the unaccompanied climber. The triumph of helping one another into a tree is a binding experience, and I like nothing better than sharing a common branch with a good friend. Yet there is something sacred about being solitary in a tree top. On my own I'm more likely to escape detection, whether by man below or beast above, and there is no compromise over which branch to choose or how far to climb. Dissecting life's problems with an airborne friend is a fine form of counselling, but the same can be said of a tree-unto-yourself, where there is no need to have the raw experience affirmed by another. Robert Louis Stevenson wrote of walking: 'You should be able to stop and go on, and follow this way or that, as the freak takes you; and because you must have your own pace.' I have often followed 'the freak' into the trees, reliant on no other agenda but my own.

I do not want this to be a technical manual. The decision to climb a tree is spontaneous and every encounter different. Rather than laying down a set of instructions, below are a few aerial insights picked up along the way.

One of the principal advantages of climbing trees over rock or ice is that a straight drop rarely confronts the climber. Unlike clinging to a cliff face, a latticework of branches intervenes between you and the ground, offering a real (or imaginary) safety net. In high summer the leaves of a tree obscure the earth below, lessening our exposure to vertical falls. The ground is glimpsed but, climbing close to the trunk, a ready anchor is always to hand.

Use the natural geometry of the tree to aid your passage. Branchless sections often provide other means of ascent, burrs for leverage or a woodpecker's hole, and some species have bark sufficiently hard and fissured to act as a hold in its own right. The way is not always obvious and few trees grow straight. In the course of a single ascent sloped stairways can transform into vertiginous overhangs. The climber must adjust to their warp and weft.

Exploring uninhibited by surplus clothing and gear is an essential freedom. You need nothing more advanced than the skin you were born in, and there are plenty of handy nooks for depositing briefcases and handbags on the way up. To further blend with a new environment, shades of grey and green lend camouflage to the climber, distancing the city below.

There are many advantages to climbing trees in bare feet. We were all born with splayed toes, perfect for balancing on branches, but our parents' insistence on stuffing infant feet into footwear undid this great gift, narrowing digits and flattening arches. A short stint of baring your soles to the elements and the old connection between skin and bark can be re-forged. Adopt a kind of 'four-hands' philosophy – our ape forebears retained opposable toes on their feet for good reason – and remember that the lighter you climb the further you'll go.

Climbing bare-footed is an altogether more immersive experience. Where shoes divorce you from the tree, skin attunes you to the feel of different types of bark and is well worth the odd stubbed toe or splinter. In wet weather a rubber heel can send you sprawling to the ground, and bare feet do less damage to the trees themselves. Sap is a wonderful natural glue and before long your naked feet will stick to bark like a gecko to a wall. If you must wear shoes in order to feel your toes in the depths of winter, don't try shimmying up a trunk in a pair of snakeskin brogues. The espadrilles once used by pioneering rock climbers are an ideal compromise. With these you can judge the camber of a branch and still avoid slipping off.

Remember to be wary of dogs. Have you ever seen the way a spaniel watches a squirrel? To the canine race, tree climbers are objects of rabid fascination, legs dangling appetisingly from on high like a line of sausages above a butcher's counter. Often I've crouched, paralysed on the groundmost branch of a tree, with ferocious terriers circling below, baying for my blood.

Climbers can also become predatory themselves. Watching people from the vantage of a branch leads one to adopt a hunter's disposition; a feeling of omniscience arising from seeing all and yet remaining unobserved. One summer's evening in Victoria Park, I found myself descending a pine after sundown. Nearing the bottom, I spotted a glowing cherry through the branches – two teenage boys sharing a joint at the tree's foot. I waited in silence for them to finish and leave. After ten minutes, when they showed no signs of moving on, my patience wore thin. In spite of the very real danger of sending them both into cardiac arrest I sprung from my branch and flew the remaining ten feet to the ground. Two priceless screams rent the silence of the park and the boys fled in opposite directions, so fast that I never saw their faces. In my vainer moments I hope they still talk of the devil that dropped from the sky.

Whiling away an hour or two in a tree top, other awkward confrontations can await the climber on descent. I have gate-crashed picnics, ball games and baby showers, arriving like an angel of ill omen from above. Epithets given me on such occasions have ranged from 'It's a fucking monkey' to 'Call the police.' These encounters are a necessary hazard of exploring the high land above London.

The more we climb, the easier it is to envy those animals better suited to the trees. Watch a squirrel sprint across the high bridge of a branch before leaping with gay abandon over a bottomless drop. Observe songbirds, alighting sound-lessly on the upper reaches while you sweat through a maze of branches below. We can spend many wasted hours mourn-ing the loss of our primate dexterity, those biaxial ball-and-socket wrist joints and elongated arms with which we might climb higher and farther. But consider the less fortunate members of the animal kingdom, those poor beasts with no prospect of ever attaining the emerald heights. The horse, the hippo, the humble cow; what hope have these of escaping their earthbound condition?

Above all, wear your scars with pride. Nothing commends a person like a jacket torn at the elbow or trousers greened at the knee. Bruises and cuts from the whip of high branches are badges of honour to parade among well-tailored ground dwellers. Turning in after a day exploring the city's trees, I once found my entire buttocks covered in a constellation of savage bites. I was eager to know what poor invertebrate had been stirred into such a frenzy of retribution. On another occasion, sitting down to a meal in a Greenwich pub, a cedar cone dropped from my hair into my neighbour's pint. This wonderful specimen had attached itself to my crop by means of some highly adhesive sap. Although forced to swap my untouched lager for his now somewhat resinous beer, I was immensely pleased that a token of the day's adventures had followed me back to earth. Stepping into a beech, cedar or pine brings us closer to nature than a thousand safaris, and has as much to teach us as an entire zoo viewed through Perspex panels.

A Warning to the Curious

Bonae actionis uir, incautius in arborem ascendens deciderat deorsum, et, contrito corpore. (A worthy man, having incautiously mounted a tree, had fallen down, and died from the bruise.)

Life of Cuthbert, Bede

In many ways you are never safer than when up a tree. The moment you climb into one you remove yourself from many of the city's everyday dangers. You are, for instance, unlikely to be mugged at altitude. Pickpockets operate far below and, generally speaking, haven't hung out in trees since the high-wayman's heyday. You'd be equally unfortunate to be hit by the number 91 from Crouch End, the five o'clock from

Waterloo or a lycra-clad cyclist with a death wish. Tourist scrums, crowded streets, screaming schoolchildren: many of a city's most frightening phenomena are confined to ground level.

This is not to say that trees are without their inherent dangers. What follows is some friendly advice, most of which is common sense. I want to encourage people to climb, but to do so knowing their own limits and those of the tree. The joy of exploring a city's canopy is too precious to throw under the health and safety steam-roller; climbing trees involves a managed risk and, with due care, we need not fall to an early grave.

It is easy to forget that what goes up must come down. In a fit of cloud-chasing exuberance you might shoot up a tree paying little, if any, attention to your return journey. It is always harder to descend a tree; instead of springing up off bended knee you are lowering yourself on tired arms, while blindly feeling for footholds. Sitting pretty on a tree top, you might be sky high with confidence. Look down between your knees and this momentary elation can swiftly change to crippling fear. However high you climb, always remember the way back.

On emerging at the top of a tree you might get the urge to jump and shout, wave frantically and generally draw attention to yourself in any manner possible. When confronted with a panoramic view of the city and a host of tiny people wandering far below, the human ego is prone to inflate to regal proportions. I call this 'king-of-the-castle complex' and strongly discourage it. Not only does such showboating distract from the important task of balancing on a branch, but you are disrespecting the noble practice of climbing trees. If you had lived in prehistory any large passing predator would have instantly devoured you. In medieval times bored archers might have used you for target practice. Today people will probably just think you're a jerk. There's a lot to be said for silent appreciation.

Remember to take a friend, at least to begin with. Exploring with a companion not only drastically expands your climbing remit, as outlined in the previous section, but also provides you with a handy insurance policy. In the unlikely event of falling from on high and injuring yourself, it's vital to have someone on hand to be a hero and help out. Lying at the bottom of a tree alone and in pain is not advised; you will only attract the attention of passing vultures.

Climbing trees is sadly no longer a national pastime, and in the city it's a rare sight. Because of this, park authorities and other powers-that-be might show surprise at finding you dangling from a branch. There is no natural law that prevents humans from climbing trees but there are a fair few man-made ones. Many of these lie open to interpretation but, even so, you may not have an inalienable right to be in your chosen tree. Be polite and find another if needs be.

When in the canopy try to resist taking endless reams of photographs. Confining the sum total of your experience to the eye hole of a camera creates memories more unreliable than your own. The camera becomes the moment itself and the joy of the climb is forgotten.

The trees themselves deserve due veneration; they've all lived here longer than you. Ancients that have survived many centuries of city life should be allowed to retire gracefully in old age without the strain of climbers on their world-weary branches.

The trees profiled in this book are mature specimens. All are sturdy plants and, if treated with respect, should not suffer from your passage from root to tip. When exploring other trees to climb, it's best to avoid those that are not yet fully grown. Rather than kill a young sapling, chart its growth over the years and return to climb it when you are both older and wiser.

Trees are host to intricate ecosystems with thousands of dependants. One of the delights of perching in tree tops is meeting a cornucopia of wildlife in the heart of the city, and your attention to detail is sharpened by focusing on every branch you climb. Bark-coloured beetles, lime-green aphids and tree-dwelling spiders cross your path. My former arach-nophobia was overcome by an encounter in a horse chestnut, a large spider crossing my arm as I clung to a high branch, giving me the option of putting up with it or breaking a leg.

Many of these creatures are easily disturbed, however, and won't take kindly to your trespassing. Squirrels give as good as they get, but other more fragile occupants should be avoided. Nesting birds are particularly vulnerable and, if you're climbing in spring, try to give a newly built nest a wide berth. Imagine if you had flown a thousand miles, spent a week courting the love of your life and persuaded her to bear your children, only for your entire home and progeny to be crushed by a climber's clumsy foot.

As you ascend, new shoots may try to blind you or impale your armpits, but avoid breaking off healthy limbs just because they stand in your way. Trees don't always submit to your will; a sprung branch or a slippery foothold might suddenly cast you to the ground. By climbing close to the trunk you give instinct a chance to save you from a fall, your limbs latching onto this dependable mast.

Nearly all trees carry deadwood. The seasoned climber is like a doctor with a stethoscope or an old tracker tapping the branches one by one as they go. Look for the outward signs: an absence of leaves, peeling bark or a difference in shade. The necrosis of a tree limb is not always obvious, so test each rung of the ladder as you travel up the trunk. Casting deadwood onto an unsuspecting head far below is like throwing a spear at someone from the third floor of an office block; equally, being knocked cold by a phone falling from a pocket is grounds for litigation. Take care when descending a tree that you don't arrive to find a corpse at its foot.

Keep an eye on the elements. Nothing ruffles the machine of the city like a strong south-westerly. Try to avoid climbing high branches on windy days as they come under strain when bending in a gale. Leaves scatter, branches snap, and whole trees are uprooted. A sudden gust might unseat you from a perch and, unless you catch a miraculous thermal, it will be a long tumble to earth. What appears sturdy from the ground might not cope with your added weight. Don't risk damage to branch or bone; batten down the hatches and wait until there's a lull.

Never climb beyond your comfort zone. If you find yourself twenty feet up a tree with your legs frozen, your confidence evaporating and your palms wet with sweat, climb down. Involuntary tree-hugging, through sheer fear not devotion, has nothing to recommend it. Remember, you are taking your life in your own hands, so value it accordingly.

Climbing trees is the antithesis of cotton-wool conservation; it is wilful engagement with nature rather than careful avoidance. We must not develop into a generation stapling 'Keep off' signs to every trunk, no longer knowing the names of the trees we're trying to protect. If we fail to connect with nature in a visceral way, a day will come when we are only capable of feeding squirrels store-bought nuts from our car window. The seminal step of reaching for that first branch turns scenery we take for granted into a living companion. The experience of climbing trees, and the curiosity it engenders, outweighs any damage done.

Canals & Rivers

London's skin is deeply sewn with watercourses, though many now conduct silent passage underground. The once mighty River Fleet runs invisible beneath office blocks, and the noble Westbourne is piped under London, confined to the ignominy of an iron tube. Like the roots of the trees, rivers have hidden subterranean capillaries, channelled and culverted beneath the modern city. London buried its waterways when they became a hindrance, and long gone are the days when we might have paddled from our front door to the corner shop. The rivers have become mass sewers, and tributaries that once served as transport links now ferry human effluent and the floating fat of restaurant and home.

Trapped and ignored, it is easy to suppose that, like the tree falling unheard in the forest, if a river flows unseen it has ceased to really flow at all. Yet these waterways are older than the city – older than England even. While their springs still flow, a thousand years interred is a fleeting moment in the life of a river. They surface in secret, running in concrete channels or narrow ditches, and a line of trees is the surest way to trace their covert passage. Where there's water there will grow life, even if that same water is choked with plastic bags, shopping trolleys and sunken glass. It's astonishing what a city's trees are prepared to drink, filtering polluted water and sending scavenged nutrients up into their crowns.

There is a strong compulsion to climb trees over water. Drawn to long branches above rivers and canals, we are imbued with a misplaced confidence, something in the brain associating water with soft landings and summers past. Inner-city streams conceal submerged dangers and still pools stagnate, but these are superficial deterrents. A tree overhanging the current combines the two fundamentals of wood and water, an elemental landscape in the midst of the man-made. These mesmeric haunts tempt the climber like few other urban spaces.

Perched over water, whether in the arms of a weeping willow or a straight-backed alder, networks of branch and leaf reflect upwards, enshrining the climber in a double image of the tree. The play of shadows and light hypnotises the most care-worn commuter as the water wages an endless battle to lick the city clean.

All London's streams flow into the wide blue artery of the Thames. Look at a satellite image of the city – snaking lines of trees hug the great river's bends, clinging to the water's edge as if trying to escape the metropolis altogether. Some of these are being toppled by riverside development, while others stand proud, like the uninterrupted march of London planes that edges the river from Blackfriars to Fulham. Climbing branches over the Thames we hang over the heart of the city and, if we listen closely, a rare natural sound can be heard – running water.

Canals, brooks and creeks offer an alternative environment, tight channels shaded by trees whose roots thread the water like long white eels. The Thames forms an abrupt gulf between north and south, while these smaller, circumscribed rivers are fissures in suburbia, boundaries crossed by irregular bridges but numberless branches. Many species of tree crowd the long, empty stretches of their straight-sided banks.

When storms lash the city the old waterways show their wrath, heavy rainfall swelling their channels and leaking into our streets, bubbling over manholes and seeping through brick and mortar. Sometimes I long for London's waters to burst their artificial bonds, purging themselves of their sordid cargo and making islands of bank-side trees. J. G. Ballard imagines such a future in *A Drowned World*, where the city lies buried in silt beneath a deep lagoon and a primordial hierarchy has re-established itself, rampant plants colonising the stairwells of tower blocks. Floating over a street still visible sixty feet below the water's surface, the narrator describes the sunken lines of London's buildings, 'like a reflection in a lake that had somehow lost its original'. Suspended on the long arm of a London plane or in the tresses of a willow, it would be easy to forget a city ever existed on these banks.

Waterside trees are prime lookouts, places to watch canal boats, Thames Clippers, and the tide of objects lost to London's current. Whether clutching a high branch over the river or perching above a creek, we enact a two-fold escape, climbing off the ground and then leaving the land altogether. Traversing branches over water allows us to cast off in our imagination; the current takes us with it on a journey, floating past long rows of riverside houses, shipyards and factories, beside green fields and long sandbars and then out into the open ocean. The climber is like lost timber, fallen from the deck of a container ship and drifting for a thousand miles.

Brothers in arms, Bishop's Park

Platanus × acerifolia/London plane & Ilex aquifolium/ Common holly

An avenue of London planes runs along the riverside at Bishop's Park. With their branches curling over the path, you walk under the arms of a cheering crowd. In season, great curtains of leaves cascade over the embankment wall, seeming to stretch out towards the river. Where these branches join the trees, perfect saddles are formed for the climber.

One of these planes shares its soil with a holly. Hollies are well adapted to thrive in shadow and this one has made a deep impression, stiff branches embedded in the side of its overlord. I use the holly as a mast to step up into the plane, taking a seat in the elbow where the two cross. Beneath me is the freckled wood of one; all around and above the leaves of the other.

At this height the holly's leaves are smooth, not spined, safe from browsing animals, although the only passing threat is an overweight Labrador. Shuffling along towards the river, I find that a holly branch has crossed the plane, rubbing up against it. The branch shifts in the wind, its underside like a flat tyre from the friction.

Beyond the footpath I edge out over the wall and across the long drop down to the river. The tide is out and the sand exposed, a beach littered with lumps of stone from the wall and a scattering of flotsam. What looks like an anchor lies half-buried in the mud. Other pieces of rusted metal could be forgotten treasure or discarded scaffolding; near the waterline the clay pipes of Victorian London are a scattering of white shards, roll-ups from another era.

A crow pecks on the foreshore at a flash of silver – foil or a bottletop – while a black-headed gull dive-bombs it from above. Leaves drift down the river and I make a promise to return in autumn, when the plane will shed its burden of broad leaves to make an armada on the water.

Retreating to the landward side of the tree, I see the branches are covered in lichen and the wood has a curious pitted appearance, whole sections with fossil-like indentations where the bark has flaked away. I climb higher and lean my back against the trunk. On the opposite bank the London

Rowing Club's slipway is jostled with cars parked at steep angles to the water, only their hand brakes saving them from immersion. Out on the wind-ruffled river, four women pull hard against the waves in a yellow scull.

The Helping Hand, Regent's Canal
Populus alba/White poplar

Standing in a narrow corridor of grass by the canal in Mile End Park are two poplars. Behind them the single chimney of a Victorian brick kiln rises above a wall of graffiti. The chimney is mirrored in the canal's green water, and drifting clouds join it in the depths.

The dried grass beneath the southernmost poplar swarms thick with crickets, a raucous mating song in the July heat wave. There exists a city all of its own in the shade of the tree, replete with ring roads and intersections among the roots. As I step into the shade, the building site beyond the grass fades to a dull rumble under the canopy's thrall.

I stand on a fairy ring of carved logs at its base, staring up at the cut-diamond patterns that decorate the bark. One great suckering root passes between my feet – I can almost feel the tree's thirst.

The upsweep of branches above me ends in great clusters of leaves, their contrasting sides of green and white giving a sense of motion, even without a breath of wind. I try to flat-foot up the poplar's slope and retreat dispirited, having moments before fallen from the first branches of another

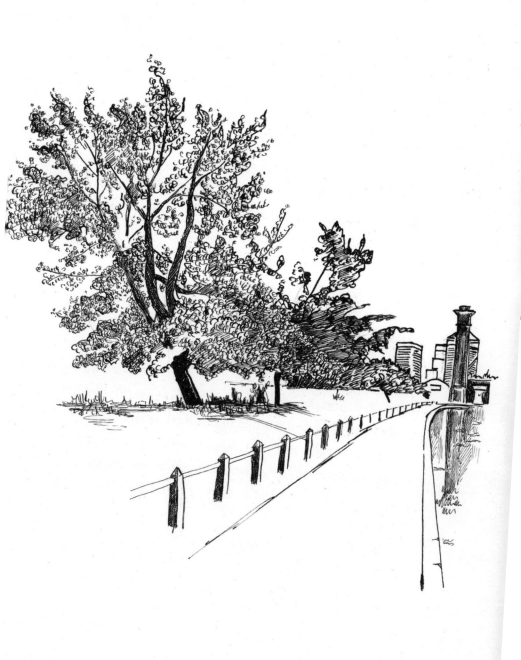

close to Limehouse Basin. Drenched in sweat, I begin to question the merits of climbing in thirty-degree heat.

Then an angel appears on the tow path, a man in a hi-vis jacket carrying a spade in one hand and a lunch bag in the other. He watches me repeatedly sliding down the trunk, then hops the railing and walks over. I turn, expecting some kind of mockery, but instead he drops the spade and asks, 'Need a leg-up?' This remains the sole occasion I've been helped into a tree by a total stranger.

Up in the bole, hoverflies molest my hair as I shuffle out along the length of a branch until I too am hovering, ten feet above the canal. Higher tiers of leaves protect my scalp from the sun, but I still have to fight the temptation to dive into the water. A solitary condom drifts past languidly, and the urge evaporates.

A black crow alights ahead of me on the branch. Perched unmoving on the poplar's white skin, it looks like a solitary chess piece. Beneath it, *Water Rat* – a canal boat – glides by and the woman at the helm waves up at me.

On my way down I defrock the poplar of a plastic bag. Returning to the tow path, I stagger to the Palm Tree pub, a precious oasis in a landscape levelled by the Blitz.

The Hideout, Beverley Brook
Fraxinus excelsior/Common ash

Wandering away from the riverbank in Putney, I find a small stream that strikes out across Barnes Common, wrapped around by a protective hedge of sycamore, oak, willow and ash.

Birds call everywhere along the brook and broken tree limbs twist in the wind, creaking loudly. The stream is surprisingly clear and, aside from a couple of beer cans, no rubbish floats along its course. The path I follow is bordered by blackberry bushes and great stands of nettles; in among these a St George's Cross has been spray-painted onto the flank of a young sycamore, an unwilling patriot.

Further on, past a bridge that leads onto Putney Heath, a magnificent dark oak rises, stag-headed, with huge white coils of dead ivy wrapped around its trunk. The tree seems half-suffocated and bent out of shape by this creeping garrotte. The ivy's dead hair is deeply cobwebbed and I wonder what kind of arachnids haunt the maze. At its base an orange ring has been daubed. Perhaps this is a mark of death and the oak has been condemned to be felled. It seems an unnecessary fate; away from the dead branch tips, leaves are sprouting from the tree's thick limbs.

I break out into Rocks Lane Field and then back to the treeline where the brook lies concealed. Stepping into a hidden clearing, the bankside is a warren of exposed roots. I climb an ash straight as a flagpole to get a better view of this intricate carpet. Below, the brook is fast-flowing back out to the river and the sea, and the sandy bottom is yellow in the afternoon sun. Two seagulls wheel overhead before turning east.

This secluded haven is the perfect schoolboy's hangout, a place to smoke stolen cigarettes and play cards. Where the brook disappears under Rocks Lane it's worth turning south behind the adjacent tennis courts to explore the remains of the Old Barnes Common Cemetery. In among a host of beheaded angels and fallen crosses is a stand of tall yew trees, shedding their poisonous crop of leaves on the dear departed.

The Old Mill, Ravensbourne River

Fagus sylvatica 'Purpurea'/Copper beech

Crossing over the bridge from Coldbath Street Estate, I catch my first sight of the Ravensbourne. Although it passes through the arse end of Deptford Creek on every tide, the river runs clear in a high-walled channel through Brookmill Park. Alongside, the tracks of the Docklands Light Railway hug the embankment on their way south.

I follow a path along the bank and pass a mighty three-pronged plane rising from a lawn by the playground. The fat bole has something stuffed into a crevice at head height. Curious, I walk over to find a tree fungus spreading inside the trunk like foam filler.

At the north end of Brookmill stands a copper beech, hard by the riverside. I grab the lowest branch and struggle clockwise around the trunk, before lifting myself through a tangle of limbs. Higher up, a curling horn of a branch provides a useful hook to rest on.

The river seen from the air seems low in its concrete channel, running back towards the Thames. Lumps of wall

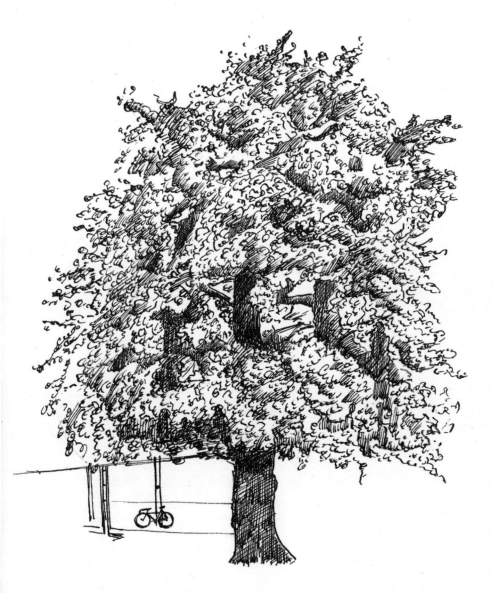

from some bygone structure sit deep in the silt, and ripples appear around them, dragging against the current. On the far side I glimpse the red-brick vault of the James Engine House through the leaves, an imposing Victorian pumping station.

Brookmill's ornamental gardens fan out to the west. The herringbone brick paths run towards a round pool with a fountain at its centre, the water conceivably drawn from the river itself. The park is deserted and no one sits on the red tubular benches that look like the requisitioned hand rails of old Central Line carriages.

Climbing as far as the branches will permit, I find an arcane symbol hacked with a knife into the uppermost part of the trunk. The pattern is impossible to decipher, more hieroglyph than 21st-century tag. I wonder how long it's been here and whether this old scar has shifted with time, the bark contorting in its annual growth cycle. Lichen prolifer- ates where the blade incised the tree, colouring the hewn bark a gaudy yellow.

Descending, I place one hand in a kind of double arch in the wood, one inverted on top of the other like the famous

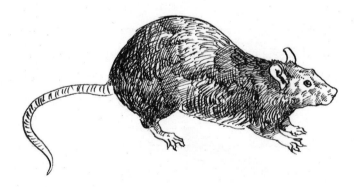

scissor divide in Wells Cathedral. The interior of the beech is a labyrinth and I slip back to the ground as if through a ball of wire mesh. As I retrace my steps along the bank two morbidly obese rats cross my path. They bob out of sight behind a fence, off to pay homage to their king.

The Crow's Nest, King Edward VII Memorial Park
Alnus glutinosa/Common alder

In Shadwell one winter's evening before sundown I find a lofty alder by the riverbank. Dwelling in a corner of the King Edward Memorial Park, the tree borders the Thameside walkway and its roots ply the river water itself, seeping through the mortar of the embankment wall.

Ducking behind the park bandstand and a row of shrubs, I pause at the alder's foot. A single long branch curls out over my head and I follow it to the point where it strays closest to the ground. I leap to catch it, and a desperate arm wrestle with the tree ensues. Climbing hand over hand, I try to swing a leg over the branch, finally gaining the relief of the trunk.

The bark above me is covered by a black film, the residue of the dual carriageway that thunders north of the park. As I climb, the river plays out between bare branches. The last light burnishes the water silver and sets small fires in the windows of Dockland towers.

Soon the ground has become nothing more than a glimpse of shadow, and the view is opening on all sides. I pass two

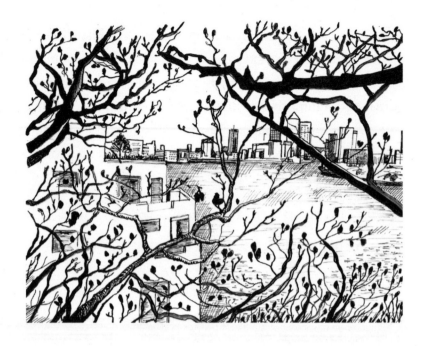

bird boxes pinned to the trunk, then draw level with the highest balcony of a riverside block of flats. Resting beneath the last branch, I imagine myself the lookout on a tall ship. Perched here it's easy to indulge in maritime fantasies, replacing passing Thames Clippers with the steamboats of yesteryear and the clear evening with a thick morning smog. The alder shifts beneath me, a rolling ship heavy with foreign cargo. I imagine sailing out to sea, perhaps in the company of Conrad. 'We live in the flicker – may it last as long as the old earth keeps rolling!' So speaks Marlow, afloat on the Thames in the opening chapter of *Heart of Darkness*. He refers to the passing ages of London, the brief moments of civilisation between long years of wilderness. From the tree top the climber can envisage a different landscape, composed of nothing more than marsh.

I turn west, and the fantasy evaporates; the megaliths of Bishopsgate stalk the skyline and the Gherkin seems close enough to reach out and polish. Descending from my panoramic seat, I glimpse a commuter crossing the park, waving with one hand, a phone in the other. From this vantage all human gestures seem exaggerated and the man is just another player in the pantomime.

The Sidewinder, Hertford Union Canal
Quercus cerris/Turkey oak

Drizzle tries to pockmark the canal, a greasy surface film repelling the rain. As I tramp along the tow path, everything seems to bleed into the water. Behind the iron railings bounding the canal, tall trees stalk the fringe of Victoria Park: planes, willows and horse chestnuts. They stand to attention, upright and aloof, offering not one branch to the waterside.

I turn back at a bridge with 'Arse' scrawled across the arch in lollipop red, before catching sight of a great crossbar of a tree, a large oak growing at an acute angle to the ground. I hop the fence to take a closer look.

The climb is straightforward but the rain has rendered the bark black and slippery, and the angle steepens as I ascend. The oak's rough contours create just enough friction to cling on, a good choice for a wet day. I slither up like a snail, chest to the tree, terrified of spinning under the sodden trunk and falling on my back.

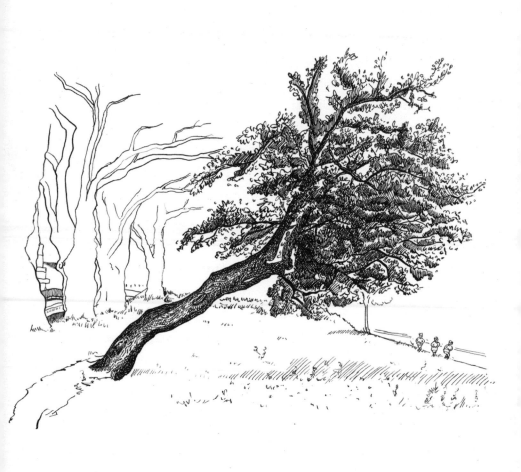

Reaching the stunted canopy, I am wearing a merman's clothing, a dark green lather covering my hands and jeans. The oak's branches form a square border beneath my feet, perfectly framing a patch of grass twenty feet below. Level with my nose, a bunch of acorns hangs between the leaves; their deep cups are covered with overlapping scales, a hallmark of the Turkey oak.

Something crosses my hand and disappears into a crevice in the wood. When climbing trees I often get the sense that I've just missed their other occupants, half-seen creatures that burrow back into the trunk as my shadow crosses them. They inhabit vast sub-cities, beyond the realm of human sight and hearing.

Perched on my summit branch the angle of the tree makes me feel exposed, like being offered up on a spoon to some passing giant. Out on the water, puffs of wood smoke drift up from a line of canal boats, their owners conversing in signal plumes. A wide barge, barely contained by the channel, is pushed past by a small grey tug, jugging along with its helmsman half-asleep by the wheel. Rain begins to pool on my lap and I climb down to find my own fireside.

The Golden Fleece, Little Venice
Liriodendron tulipifera/Tulip tree

Two canals meet in Little Venice, and at their junction the clean-bordered lawn of Rembrandt Gardens drops to the water's edge. Spreading across the southern end is a tall tulip tree. At the tail end of October its notched leaves are a cascade of liquid gold, turning the tree into a glowing tower.

A pair of lovers sit acrobatically intertwined on a bench and, when their mouths are not locked, phrases like '*Amore mio*' escape. Romeo and Juliet are too busy necking to object to me climbing over them, and I wonder if they've been hired by the local council to reinforce the waterway's branding.

The crux of the climb is, as with so many trees, the first ten feet. I leap for the lowest branch and smear up the trunk

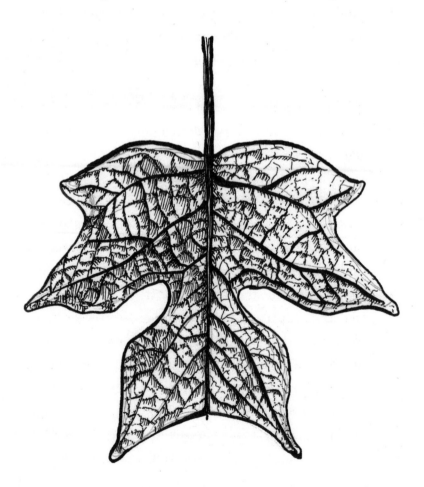

until I can hook my heel in the fork, swapping foot for hand. From the ground this manoeuvre is particularly undignified, and two girls point and laugh at me. Above, the pale-grey bark is branchless, and I have to swing out and around the tree, my knees gripping the trunk. I receive a free body scrub from this operation, a fine sand-papering of the inner thighs, and wish I had an orangutan's thick body hair to protect my flesh.

Surveying the damage, I notice my clothes have attracted a large following of green aphids. I pull a leaf towards me, the whole underside covered in their sticky, honeydew secretion. Brushing through the foliage, I have become a vehicle for legions of these insects, stuck fast on my shirt and jeans.

I continue to climb with my new congregation until the branches dwindle; back down the length of the trunk the autumnal fire of the leaves is staggering, a beacon on a grey day. Beyond this golden fleece, pedestrians pass on the far side of the canal, a mother screaming at her children for fishing with their hands in the water. The *Lionheart* and an old Thames barge with paddleboards drift idle alongside them, circumnavigating *The Lady A*, which lies at anchor. This is a mecca for the trainspotters of the water world.

Filtered through plane trees, the island in the heart of Little Venice is covered with geese and guano. The birds move in circles around a clump of weeping willows and, in the distance, a blue bridge marks the end of this avian paradise. Later, unpacking my rucksack at home, I find a single gold leaf clinging to the zip, a beautiful relic of pre-Ice Age flora.

The Tree Climber's Guide

The Double Decker, Millbank
Platanus × acerifolia/London plane

A line of generous London planes follows the river at Millbank, dropping inviting arms over the Embankment wall. Each one seems to recoil from the road, leaning into the open space overhanging the water.

The first plane that tempts me into its arms stands guard over the Millbank Millennium Pier. A thick lower branch cuts across the pavement at right angles, passing a few feet above the wall. I step onto the parapet, laced with fallen plane seed and moss, before clambering up. As I scuffle towards the trunk, my dangling feet threaten to clip passing pedestrians and I get a sour look from a man in a very fine hat. He stalks off in a huff with the air of someone whose headwear denotes high office.

Just before limb meets bole another branch shoots sideways, like a boat's tiller, and I use this to rise to my feet, climbing on up to a perch a few rungs higher. North of my armchair seat is the blank face of Millbank Tower, fifty years old and already Grade II listed. The doors never seem to close as hundreds of civil servants stream in and out. On the riverside the ferry docking station looks like something designed by a Bond villain, a multifaceted steel hulk sitting low in the water.

Exploring the rest of the avenue, I find a plane with a six-fingered summit fanning out over a bus shelter. Its southern arm rests on the river wall, bound to the parapet as if with cement. I drop my chest forward into the fork of the branches

and, once aboard, a
second arm overhead
provides a guide line to
the upper storeys.

A number 87 bus pulls up
alongside the tree. Sitting
level with the top deck,
I wave at a couple of
people looking out of the
window. One laughs
silently behind the
glass, the other
frowns and
gives me the
middle finger.

Directly
across the road,
steps lead up to
the grand portico of
Tate Britain. The
building is capped by
Britannia herself, trident in
hand and with the tree's lobed leaves ornamenting her hair.
Swinging around to a perch on the other side, I watch the
tree's lower branches being lapped by the high tide, dead
fingers washed with brackish water. I consider climbing
down an arm and dropping over the Embankment to hang
hidden from the world, a few feet above the current. The
river's sinister swirls and rapids make me think better of it.

Ophelia's Treehouse, The Bow Brook
Salix × sepulcralis/White weeping willow

On a small cutback from the Regent's Canal is a slice of turf and tarmac, with two weeping willows tumbling into the water.

Threading my way through a housing estate to the water-front, I use the railings that run alongside the canal to step up into the larger tree, the trunk twisting up under a broad crown of willow fronds and the gold-tinted leaves enclosing me on all sides.

Reaching a fork over the canal, I sit with my legs hanging above the water. A shifting light reflects on the undersides of the branches but the canal beneath lies shallow and stagnant. The 'muddy death' suffered by Ophelia, falling from a willow in Shakespeare's *Hamlet*, would be hard to replicate here. She'd have to be snagged by a shopping trolley to stand any chance of drowning.

The tree is a hybrid between the Chinese weeping willow (*Salix babylonica*) and the white willow (*Salix alba*). The quintessential riverside ornament, it has an enormous thirst to slake and large, exploratory roots. The concrete lip of the canal hems in the willow but its tendrils may well have split this underwater retainer.

I return down the trunk to find the ground below littered with nitrous oxide canisters, a magpie pecking speculatively among them. Perhaps a group of teenagers sat huddled in the willow itself, filling the canopy with laughing gas while shooting the breeze.

The Fireman's Pole, Meadowbank

Acer pseudoplatanus/Sycamore

Peeking over the north-east corner of Chelsea Bridge is a stand of diseased sycamores. The tallest of them stretches its upper branches over a lamp post topped by a golden boat, Battersea's coat of arms, but their roots lie some twenty feet below, down in the no man's land of Meadowbank.

In a pause between bands of pedestrians I hop up onto the bridge wall and put a foot into the crown of the nearest sycamore. Transferring my weight, I let go of the bridge and commit myself to dropping out of sight. This is the first time I have 'climbed' a tree in reverse, from top to bottom; beneath me the branches peter out, the trunk dropping straight to the ground like a fireman's pole. My descent is not so elegant and I trap my testicles on the way down, landing with a crackle in a mound of aluminium cans: Carlsberg Special Brew and Kestrel.

The Meadowbank is a psychogeographer's wet dream. Like Robert Maitland in J. G. Ballard's *Concrete Island*, I've fallen through a gap in the city and into a modern-day Hades, a desolate tangle of weeds and rubbish, lost beneath the Embankment and the bridge. This twilight zone is officially closed to members of the public, although access may be granted for the purpose of 'nature conservation study or fishing'. It is a strange kind of nature area, overlaid with mounds of uncollected rubbish haunted by rats, and the plant life runs wild, untamed by groundskeepers.

I walk east, my face brushed by plastic bags hanging from

the shrubs overhead; I need a machete to better navigate this underworld. Crossing a black plastic mat on a bed of soaked newspaper, I sense someone has stayed here not long ago – perhaps they are crouching nearby, watching me and wondering how to dispose of an unwelcome intruder.

How long would a corpse go undetected down here? The most compelling aspect of London's lost corners is the number of people passing in close proximity every day, yet never venturing in. A body rotting down here might go unnoticed longer than one abandoned in a Highland ditch. Only a noxious smell rising into the nostrils of a morning jogger would betray the cadaver below.

I pass along bent fencing above a brick wall, the Thames sloshing a few feet below and pigeons eyeing me warily from a line of hawthorns. Round the corner lies the gaping mouth of the Grovesnor Canal, a defunct sluice gate swarming with mallards that flee from my footsteps and make for the open river.

Scrambling up the steep bank and back to the road feels like emerging from a mildewed well bottom. I climb over the black guard rails of a small promontory set aside 'for the enjoyment of the public'. Inside is an unprepossessing concrete bench with a view of nowhere, and the gate remains securely padlocked.

The Fish Hook, River Wandle

Platanus × acerifolia/London plane

I start south on the Wandle Trail, a gravel path that hugs the riverside from Wandsworth to Croydon. Opposite the Garratt Park Allotments poplars and willows grow thick on the bank, hiding the industrial estates that hem the water in. Sporadic gaps in the trees reveal humming electrical substations and long lines of dumper trucks.

I pass along Norbury Brook, a fenced tributary filled with clumps of Canadian pondweed writhing in the current. Beyond lies the desert of Wandle Nature Meadow Park, a former sewage works turned nature reserve. The dual currents of river water and electricity run parallel, high-voltage wires emitting a hiss like rain water falling on hot coals. The river looks fit to burst and flood the open ground, creating islands of the electricity pylons.

Further down the trail at the southern end of Wandle Park, the river is bounded by a fence of fish hooks, iron spikes curled over at the top. One of these has been removed and I squeeze through the gap to get down to the riverbank. Following a line of lager cans to the foot of a London plane, I find a mass of exposed roots tumbling to the water's edge, the hollows between filled with dead leaves.

A long flaking arm stretches out across the river. The ivy on the backside of the tree is not thick enough to serve as a rope ladder but a dead spar sticks out under the branch. I pull up on this, hoping it will bear my weight, and emerge, wheezing, onto the perch.

Far out along the branch are the twisted remains of a rope swing, cut off at the knot. The whole scene feels like the echo of someone else's childhood, when the river ran with trout and no one came here to get drunk. The sky has turned purple with thundercloud and I watch a squirrel run along the river's edge, an entire foil-wrapped KitKat clenched in its jaw. Perhaps this is not his first theft, and corner shops across Merton dread his visits. I swing down from the deadwood and leave the way I came, crawling back through the fencing.

City Parks

The journalist James Bone took to the air over London in 1917, grasping the rickety cockpit of a Handley Page aeroplane. From this precarious platform of canvas and wood he looked down over the vast city beneath him. Bone's first horrified impression was 'of civilisation as a terrible sausage-machine, which received humanity and pressed it into close, red, squirmy residue'. London's inhabitants were 'lost in the smoky sea' of industry, doomed to be squeezed slowly to death. A bleak spectacle stretched away to every horizon.

Moments later, the airborne writer flew over the trees of a city park and his mood completely changed. In rhapsodic terms he celebrated the 'huge grey-green oasis among the tiles and slates', a wooded vale surrounded by a halo of pollution. He saw the city's green spaces as a promised land against the backdrop of chimneys, cranes and crowded streets.

Times have changed since Bone clung to his biplane, and the smog of London has lifted, but the parks established during the Industrial Revolution are flourishing today. Many of the city's younger green spaces owe their inception to the public park movement, started by a 19th-century collective of altruists committed to halting urban sprawl. London's parks developed into model blueprints for other cities, and space and light were introduced into overcrowded neighbourhoods.

Parks are the tree climber's bread and butter, and their most uninhibited playground. The sense of common ownership that exists in these spaces has given people licence to follow their whims, however unorthodox. Swordplay, chanting, sadomasochistic military drills – all have their place in the park pantheon. From dawn till dusk and beyond I have watched men and women conduct the private rituals of a thousand personal creeds. People retreat to the odd corners of parks with the same intent: to alleviate the soul-crushing uniformity of the city's routine.

The shade of trees also provides a hideaway for the illicit: drug dealing, public sex, taking a crap. I've never forgotten playing tennis in a park only to have every other serve punctuated by a protracted orgasm. Retrieving a stray ball I discovered the source, a couple copulating behind a swamp cypress.

For the climbing addict the plotted landscapes of the city's parks have an appeal all of their own. Trees are planted at measured intervals and in studied relation to their surroundings, free to grow to their full span away from the forest's dim light or the shadow cast by office blocks. Beech, ash and oak sprawl in this rare luxury of space. Viewed from up a tree on a clear day, branches decorate park lawns with interlaced shadows. From well-loved roosts to rarely visited heights, an immense range of climbing can be found across London's parkland.

A number of the parks explored here have more than one tree listed, while other parks have been omitted entirely – the spread of London's best perches is uneven. Some of my favourite parks lack a single decent climb; others abound with ladder-like trees.

We become insular creatures in the city and, although our local park might be as familiar as our own home, few of us explore the green spaces beyond. A park that lies under half a mile from your door may contain a trove of untrod branches.

The Divine Tree, Holland Park
Cedrus deodara/Deodar

Well-groomed men and dogs stride side by side through the green lanes of Holland Park. When I enter through the

Abbotsbury Road gate, two bejewelled octogenarians march past with their pugs on opposite sides of the path. The dogs catch sight of one another and pull their reluctant owners together, powerless against the attracting magnets of randy toy dogs.

The north end of the park is heavily wooded, its tall copses enclosed behind iron guard rails. I hug these perimeter fences, eagerly trying to catch sight of any climbable trees within. Before long the path emerges into the Japanese Kyoto Garden. A large band of sugar-high school children have been unleashed on this idyllic retreat; manicured shrubs and golden carp recoil from their screams.

Near to the North Lawn I pass under a deodar and feel its weeping branches brush my shoulder. Native to the steep slopes of the Himalaya, this cedar is descended from on high; the Latin *deodara* means 'timber of the Gods'. Standing at the tree's foot, its roots bulge like muscles beneath it, creating long ripples in the soil.

I wait for a Dacia with 'Park Police' stamped on its flank to roll by before stepping up into the low-hanging branches. They run smooth and straight, and once in among them an odour of wet spice seeps into the close air beneath the canopy. The tree's foliage forms a heavy velvet drapery, like the stage curtains of the nearby Holland Park opera; climb the cedar during the season and it's possible to eavesdrop on open-air performances. The wind catches a branch and a whorl of needles drapes my forehead with a long, green fringe.

The surrounding park is thick with parakeets, and their short bursts of manic laughter mock me as I climb higher. An

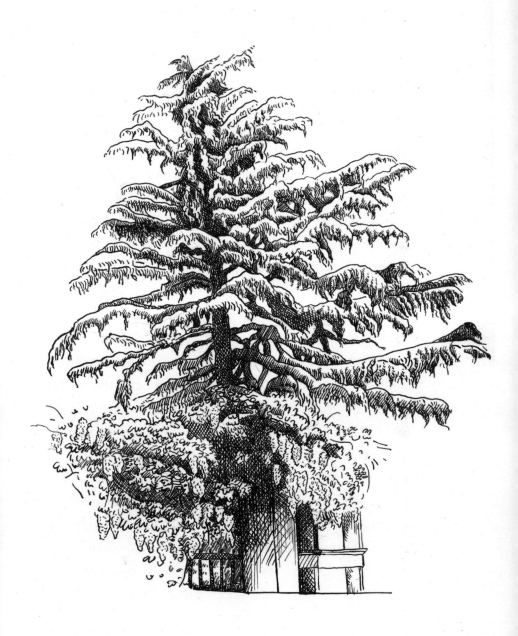

estimated fifty thousand of these birds now live wild in Britain, although their origin is shrouded in mystery – one theory blames Jimi Hendrix for releasing the first breeding pair.

In the middle branches of the deodar the remains of a yellow security tape are tied to a limb, the last time the tree was co-opted into public service. Pocketing this plastic snake, I climb another five feet to a perch with a window on the park below. From here a chocolate-box view of the Dutch Garden unfolds, tulips in every conceivable shade. I spot a contender for London's saddest statue, a miserable cloaked figure grimacing from his niche in the garden wall.

Opposite the deodar is a beautiful copper beech inter-twined with a giant wisteria that climbs up from the brick wall into its crown. The wisteria's pale-purple flowers weave through the russet leaves. On the north side of the tree a small girl stands practising with a bow and arrow in a clear-ing, firing at a tennis ball in the crook of a horse chestnut. Her father watches with obvious pride, the scene posed like a page from a medieval manuscript. At my back rise the remnants of Holland House, hit by twenty-two incendiary bombs one long night in September 1940. I imagine this landscape on fire, liquid flames engulfing tree roots, and descend the deodar in search of a drink.

The Kraken, Clissold Park
Aesculus hippocastanum/Horse chestnut

Entering Clissold Park from the south, I pass the goat sanctuary where the sole occupant has his head pressed to a wall. Beyond, a parade of venerable horse chestnuts marches across the green, as old as the park itself.

One tree drifts like an octopus above the sea floor, its lower branches extending great tentacles and shading the ground with seven-fingered leaf clusters. A little apart from the main trunk, a sucker erupts like Nessie from the park lawn, a monster wading through the grass, intent on rampaging into central London.

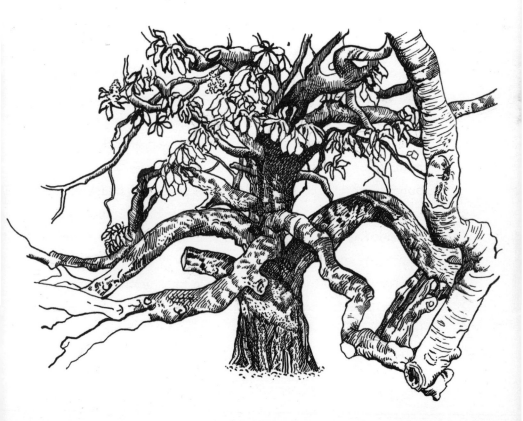

This is the perfect climbing tree: wrought by two centuries of good London living, its sinuous spread presents any number of routes into the canopy. The easiest of these is a branch that splits in two at its tip, like the wishbone of a chicken. Placing a hand on each prong at chest height, I swing both legs into the joint. Once up on the bridge it is broad enough for me to stand and walk up towards the trunk.

If the width of the branches isn't climbing aid enough, knuckles sprout from mid-limb like vertebrae trapped beneath the bark. I use these for balance and hoist myself higher. Reaching the trunk, I turn and look back at the tree's awesome spread. Twenty friends could happily picnic in the lower branches alone.

Unlike almost every other tree in this book, I've often found fellow climbers in its branches. The paths of ascent are too many and too obvious, and the tree exerts a magnetic pull on passers-by. The horse chestnut is well loved, even if some of its devotees have a strange way of showing it; on my last visit Coke cans lay side by side with blossom in the tree's bole.

Some visitors have left their mark with paint or knife. If you climb to the tree's highest fork and look up into the shrouded sky overhead, someone's initials are etched on a thin limb hanging over a drop of forty feet. The tree might not have agreed to this tattoo but it's hard not to admire the climber's dedication. Graffiti at ground level is an eyesore but bark marked at altitude carries with it an aura of conquest.

The horse chestnut is surrounded by other majestic contemporaries. Don't miss its squat neighbour to the east, a tree with a crown like the spread wings of an eagle or the centre-parting of a bad wig.

The Cracked Ash, Victoria Park
Fraxinus excelsior/Common ash

On the north-eastern corner of Victoria Park's boating lake a curving trail follows the shore to meet a bandstand supported by varnished tree trunks. In the open field beyond, and bordering the formal gardens, stands a thick ash, a resident here since the 1850s.

From a distance the ash looks the wrong shape to scale. The branches sprout upwards from a broad trunk like a giant broccoli, and there are no low-hanging holds. On closer inspection the rough bark provides the way up, a series of rock-hard fissures deep enough to wedge fingers into.

The ascent is a rock climber's dream. Conquering the cliff-like trunk requires counter-balance, and I lean back with hands and feet, pivoting against my own body weight. I hang on the face then stretch to sink a fist in a nook in the bole.

Sitting in the tree's heart and drawing breath, I see that both of my bare feet have been cut by the bark's grooves. To add insult to injury, my shirt receives a direct hit from a magpie dancing in the tree top, a purple-flecked deposit with a berry stone at its centre. The culprit continues to victory-

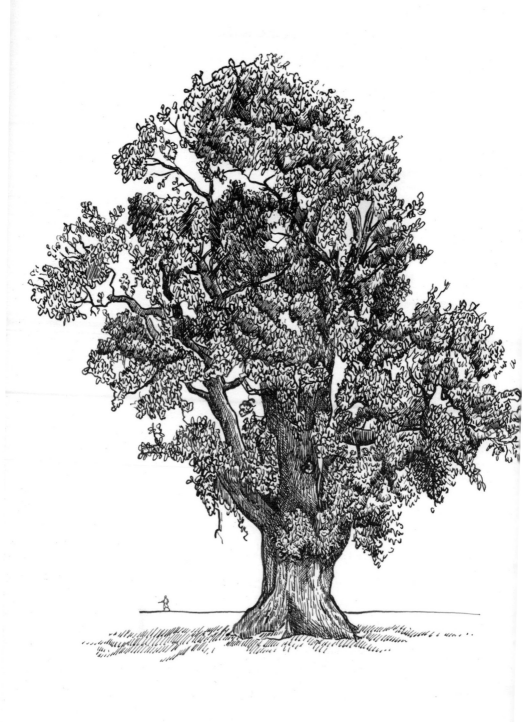

hop across the crown, and the old superstition that bird shit on the shoulder signals good luck gives me scant consolation.

I move on up the sharp curve of the western arm and find a flat seat where I can lodge myself, feet overhanging the park. All around me ash leaves blow with the breeze, and my thoughts also drift at the wind's mercy.

The tree has an airy interior, with light, shifting foliage that allows the sun to fall through to my seat. Looking at this broad spread I can believe in the ash of Norse legend, Yggdrasil, whose branches supported the heavens and whose roots ploughed down to hell.

Spend ten minutes aloft in this ash and a kaleidoscope of London life passes by; speed-walkers, marathon men, dogs, drunks, skaters, prams, all these attest to the nickname, 'the People's Park'. It's a cauldron of comings and goings. A plaintive bark from the base of the tree reminds me that my own dog awaits my return, his Roman nose turned expectantly skyward. Reluctantly, I leave the hypnotic dome of the ash for another day.

Twin Peaks, Victoria Park
Pinus radiata/Monterey pine

Up above the model boating lake of Victoria Park are two magnificent sisters, twin pines facing each other across ground thick with their fallen needles. Side by side they look like conspirators, hiding smirks behind dark-green shrouds.

One stands ramrod straight while the other leans across, as if sharing an aerial secret with its sibling. There is a distinct Lynchian atmosphere to the scene, and I half expect to see grinning nudists dance between the trees and then vanish into the shrubbery.

Both conifers offer low branches to the climber, but the tree to the west quickly becomes an overhang, listing like a wooden Tower of Pisa. Switching to its twin, I clamber up through secure scaffolding, sticking close to the trunk and locked into a natural ladder. I pass a column of bird boxes stacked one above the other like show flats, each with a better view than the last.

Gaining height, the Docklands reveal themselves away to the south. In windows through the foliage the pyramid of One Canada Square appears and vanishes again, obscured by swaying branches. I feel deeply hidden and alone; no one passes beneath the closed circle of the tree.

Under me lie the formal gardens of Victoria Park, neat borders where dogs run with gay abandon and shit on the primroses. Beyond, open playing fields dotted with holm oaks stretch away to the eastern boundary. Somewhere, out of sight beneath curling London planes are two squat stone alcoves, the last remnants of the old London Bridge, towed over here in the 18th century and now thick with moss.

Bristowe's Oaks, Brockwell Park
Quercus robur/*English oak*

A twisting English oak stands in a grove enclosed by dead-wood, a ring of fallen logs like the remains of a stone circle. Nearby, the sound of laughter leaks out of the park lido, an Art Deco beach in the heart of south London.

I step up into the tree using an old stump under the fork. The seasoned bark is a useful prop and hard, armoured ridges aid my grip. Straddling wide branches, I ascend haphazardly as if clambering over a turnstile. After much doubling back on myself I reach a perfect level perch and wish I'd brought a book; this is a tree in which to spend the whole day idling.

English oak seems to age in a more human way than other trees. Placing my hand on the bark, I feel the fissured skin and set wrinkles of its growth lines. A 'stag's head' of dead-wood caps the tree, hair loss for an old oak, and the broken crown is hollowed out but still handsome.

Relaxing in the tree top for a half-hour, I notice a curious rhythmic sound emanating from the middle of the grove, a bass line repeating itself over and over. Leaning down from my branch, I can just make out a bearded man in a brown smock chanting in the shadow of another tree. He continues intoning the same unintelligible words and I climb down, feeling guilty for spying on his ritual.

Walking up the rump of Brockwell Park, I come to a second oak, an evergreen on the south side of the building that straddles the hill. Thomas Bristowe, the man who finally secured this park for the people, collapsed and died here shortly after the opening ceremony in 1892, his life's work achieved. Passing under the tree, I trip on its knees, great doorstop roots standing proud above the ground. The holm oak's canopy is a broad dome, and I hold on to a crook between its branches before following a path up into the tree.

The leaves are a dark green, almost black, and rolling one between my hands it crackles like dry tinder in a fire. I close my eyes and settle down in the branches. When I open them again, a third-quarter moon has risen over the park.

Plimpton's Seat, Finsbury Park
Cedrus libani/Cedar of Lebanon

George Plimpton was a remarkable writer. A man who won fame for his 'participatory journalism', he put his body on the line in contests with professional sportsmen, from sparring with Sugar Ray Robinson to taking a pummelling as back-up quarterback for the Detroit Lions.

My thoughts turn to Plimpton as I idle in a cedar, deep in Finsbury Park. Spreading in front of me is an ocean of needles and cones, but beyond and below span the concentric ovals of the athletics ground, home to London Blitz, the city's most successful American football team. I like to think Plimpton would have taken great pleasure in climbing this tree to watch a group of men in lycra beat each other to a fleshy pulp; the perch is a grandstand ticket.

The cedar was planted in the park's old arboretum, an area peppered with other ornamental conifers. My climb requires a short but strenuous passage straight up the trunk, hooking both hands over the first bough and flat footing up the incline. A second tier is reached with an undignified scrabble over the drop, but those bold enough will be well rewarded by their effort; beyond, the tree splits and an easy set of shorter branches leads up to the summit.

The trunk ends abruptly at twenty feet, chopped straight across by a chainsaw. Rarely have I come across such a comfortable pedestal and I spend a full hour resident in the tree. Undulating plains of cedar branches stretch in every direction, like my own private lawn floating above the park, and voices drift up from the pathways below: French, Polish, Chinese, Bengali. Haringey is one of the most ethnically diverse boroughs in the city.

Finsbury Park was created on the edge of old Hornsey Wood as a permanent place of escape from the smog-bound city. The boundaries of London have long since exceeded its original green belt, but the park retains an atmosphere of evasion. It feels like a good place to run away to.

The Flagpole, Wandsworth Park
Quercus robur/English oak

Walking through Wandsworth Park in mid-December, an icy wind whisks off the Thames and barrels through the long avenue of plane trees by the bank.

Next to the playground is a tall oak, straight as an arrow and blessed with an even spread of branches from foot to tip. I climb hand over hand up this wooden ladder, stopping on the wider branches to warm my fingers.

Polished bark is evidence that the oak has attracted other climbers over the years, but today, aside from a couple wrapped up in thick scarves, the surrounding park is deserted. Higher up the tree and the climbing becomes virgin territory with no sign of human passage.

From the final branch I look down on the crazy golf course in miniature, strangely desolate without a crowd of putters on its astroturf. The river glints cold and hard through the skeletal heads of the London planes and the sun begins to dip in the west over Heathrow or Slough. The last light in Wandsworth Park seems to set the tree on fire, as if centring on the oak alone. Leaning against the trunk, and illuminated by the sunset, I can see why druids got so hung up on oak trees, bark turned to gold and leaves to flame.

I look south along the length of the Thames and think of another oak I've known, a dead Suffolk tree, seemingly held together by ivy and finally blown down by a North Sea storm. I remember climbing through its upturned roots, the inverted image of a dead giant. The roots of oaks can spread as far as three times their height. I wonder at what lies beneath the clay of Wandsworth Park.

Climbing down, a dull roar reverberates through the canopy as lorries make their way up the Putney Bridge Road and the wind lifts the tree's outspread fingers, their voice soon drowning out the traffic. Numbed by the frozen branches, I warm up in a nearby pub, The Cat's Back, where a dog at the bar sniffs my feet, perhaps surprised to find out where I've been.

The Tilted Tree, Ravenscourt Park
Quercus ilex/Holm oak

Walking up the east side of Ravenscourt Park, I come across a giant snake in the grass made from a thousand pansies. A pair of shining brogues lies beside the floral head, as if the petalled monster has just digested a passing salesman.

In a gated section of the park next to the pond a holm oak leans at a sharp angle to the ground.

Looking up from its roots, I spy a long muscular arm hanging overhead, the bark twisted like an old dishcloth. To reach this perfect picnic spot I employ the square shoulders of a good friend, stepping up onto the slope of the trunk and clutching at the great knuckle on the north side of the tree. Bringing my feet up as close to the knuckle as possible, I stand up to grasp a branch hanging down from the face. The deep, nut-brown bark of the oak is sharp as a sea cliff, so my shoes stay on. From this point it's simple to gain the crook. I reach down to give my companion a hand up and then we journey out together along the great spiral branch, before toasting our success with a tangerine.

For those taken by the charms of this evergreen oak, the upper branches of the tree can be gained by crossing its bare midriff, the gentle slope compensating for a short section without branches. The tree top affords a beautiful view south over the pond and the cedar drinking from its shallows.

Once back on the blessed ground I wander over to the two concrete ears that sit beside the playground, miniature replicas of awesome, pre-radar warning devices. I practise whispering 'Quercus ilex' into the cupped concrete a few times until I attract strange looks and move on.

The Two Towers, Ravenscourt Park
Cedrus deodara/Deodar

Following the alley from the Underground station, I spy an enormous deodar standing solitary on the west side of the park, the splayed fingers of two trunks rising high into the spring sky.

Climbing this tree is a bit like scaling a giant menorah candle. The stems and branches rise from the bole like teapot spouts and I have to wedge my ankles between them. To avoid continually doing the splits between the two trunks, I begin on the south tower and climb to the tree's mid-section before moving onto the north stem to gain the summit.

There is a well-stocked gallery of graffiti to pass on your way to the top. About thirty feet up the tree someone called Kyle decided to stop and hack out his name in five-inch letters – he must have been wielding a machete. Just below the summit are the initials 'JL', surrounded by a heart. At the time of writing the carving was fresh, showing off the clay-red colour of the cedar's cambium layer. Some of the branches have tiny, hoof-shaped markings, as if a herd of miniature horses has stampeded around their circumference.

At the top I hook an arm around the trunk and lean out to look at the view through knots of cedar cones. Across the middle of the park a cluster of church spires recedes towards the horizon where the revolving top of the BT Tower is eclipsed by my outstretched thumb. The cones at the summit have disintegrated in the wind, spreading their scales across the park and leaving bare stalks like lollipop sticks on the branches.

Three men playing football near the tree's roots punt it high into the air. The ball passes within ten feet of my face in seeming slow motion, the gold stitching visible to the naked eye, but the players following its arc don't seem to notice me.

Dismounting from the deodar, I cross over the lawn to a London plane with a curious stunted beauty, a small crown topping a trunk with a girth of nearly twenty feet. I watch a young couple lift their child into branches that must seem like a small forest to a toddler's eyes. The old plane is a magical bulwark and always has a ring of people seated at its feet.

House of Marvell, Waterlow Park

Pterocarya fraxinifolia/Caucasian wingnut

High on a north London slope, Waterlow Park is 'a garden for the gardenless', an estate gifted by its philanthropic owner to the poor of London in 1889.

The interior is a cornucopia of tree species, and I am drawn to a group of hornbeams overlooking a green gully that falls away towards central London. As I approach, a stooped man passes beneath, his metal detector swinging to and fro in haphazard appraisal of ring pulls and other buried treasure. Leaning against the largest hornbeam and looking south, I get a curious case of grounded vertigo, a feeling of slipping down the steep lawn past the ponds and out through a band of trees into the city.

I move across to a nearby bench in memory of 'Adam Shaw, Scriptwriter. A man of great courage who loved London 1963–2004'. Sitting there, I find this spare epitaph comforting, a virtue and a place giving the record of one man's life.

My quest for a climbable tree draws me away from Shaw's seat and the view down to the southern end of the park. An elderly jogger with a purple rinse flashes by in front of me for a third time. Is she conducting an endless circuit of the park? Close by a blasted oak, its trunk hollowed by fire – lightning, perhaps? – stands a wingnut tree, growing in an undisturbed corner.

Pterocarya fraxinifolia is a member of the walnut family. Comparatively rare in London, the tree's pinnate leaves can

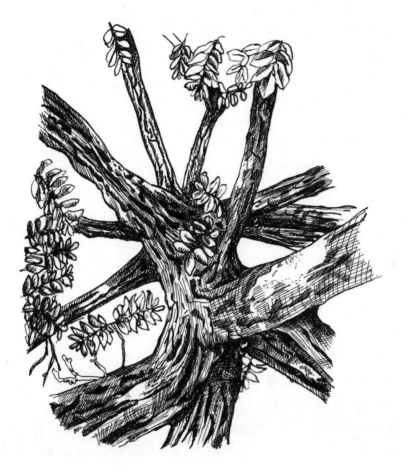

easily be mistaken for those of an ash, though they are significantly longer. The bark is covered in a sticky secretion and two jet-black spiders hurry away into its crevices. I place my left hand in a large cleft on the north side of the trunk and balance both my feet on its sloping edge. The mature wood is composed of thick flutes, excellent purchase as I reach up to grasp the lowest branch.

On reaching the top via a series of ribbed branches I look down on the roots, smooth and hard as concrete and breaking the earth around the base. Their meandering leads my eye to a line of tombstones peeking through the spring undergrowth on the border with Highgate Cemetery.

Crouched motionless in the ceiling of the tree and drowned in summer leaves, I think of the words of Andrew Marvell, the poet whose home once stood in this very park:

Annihilating all that's made
To a green Thought in a green Shade.

The Enchanted Oak, Ruskin Park
Quercus cerris/Turkey oak

The Turkey oak presides over the path close by a tiled green shelter. Easily a double centurion, born at the foot of some long-dead Londoner's garden, its germination preceded the founding of the park by over a hundred years.

The spread of the tree is enormous and seems to have been conjured straight from the pages of some Gothic horror, dark arms overshadowing the walkway that runs beneath it. The largest of these is a great beckoning finger, ensnaring anyone with a mind to climb.

When I step under the oak a woman is practising yoga at the tree's foot, alone on a black mat. I wait for her to finish before clambering up onto the extended branch, careful to avoid boarding too near the tip and placing unnecessary strain on its furthest reaches.

Timidly, I begin the long ascent to the trunk. At first I climb on all fours, ancillary branches providing leverage on the steeper section. Once on the bridge I'm forced to sit astride it, using the branch as a saddle. As I traverse its length I find the arm is a tree unto itself, as thick as the trunks of lesser specimens.

Approaching the bole, I move into the mouth of the oak, a gaping maw with two huge arms extending over my head. I feel like a fly in the jaws of a spider. Here we have the door to another world, every bit as magical as C. S. Lewis's wardrobe or J. K. Rowling's halfway station platform.

A cupped hole in the trunk above would make a brave perch but, when I peer into it, the basin is filled with rainwater from the morning's downpour. Orange stripes run along the fissures in the oak and, above, the burred trunk twists upwards; you would need all the chiropractors in London to straighten it, one wooden knot at a time.

From this vantage point I can see the cranes of nearby construction projects, backed by the intermittent whistles of South London Line trains. Down below, streams of joggers have replaced the yogi, passing in neon rainbows under the oaken bridge. Not one looks up from pounding the park dirt.

I dare not turn on the high branch, and decide to reverse the way I have come. Moving backwards along the bridge, I feel like an old carriage shunting down the rails, one sleeper at a time. Just before I drop back onto the path a bright-green aphid alights on my forearm. This last emissary from the great oak is a reminder of the other city that inhabits its crevices, tiers of insect food chains relying on its magnanimity.

The Quarterdeck, Geraldine Harmsworth Park
Platanus × *acerifolia/London plane*

I duck beneath the barrels of hundred-tonne guns guarding the doors to the Imperial War Museum. A plaque beneath their century-old frame states they are capable of firing pig-sized shells sixteen and a quarter miles. With the current orientation of their sights that would mean obliterating a large part of Potters Bar.

I abandon military history for the park's 'Ice Age Tree Trail', a journey around the thirty-four native species that recolonised Britain when the ice melted. I make it as far as a cherry tree to whose trunk a notice has been taped, advertising mulberry picking with the head gardener. Sprinting across to the potting sheds, I find I've missed the mulberries by five minutes and buy an ice cream to get over the disappointment.

A great four-armed London plane rises beside the museum's south corner. On one side of the trunk there's a small burrow in the base and a burr for a foothold. Balanced on

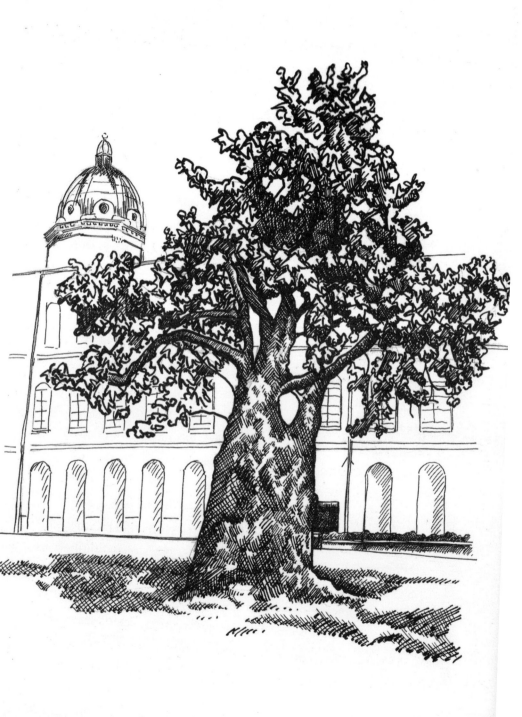

this protrusion I reach above and find the lip of the bole is a narrow ridge, perfect leverage to pull myself into the tree.

Inside, a warped throne sits between the spreading arms, the bark's mildew dappled with sunlight. I look north to where two neighbouring planes cut comic poses, squat trees with carrot-top crowns. Moving through the centre to the southern branch, I crawl halfway up to catch the afternoon sun. Below me, one of the museum's security guards paces up and down, a walkie-talkie clamped tight to his ear.

On my way out, I stop by another plane at the opposite end of the park, its trunk wrapped around with five floors of scaffolding. Sitting on the third of these in a throne made from deadwood is the artist known as Morganico. He looks down on me, wood chip in his beard, over the teeth of a large chainsaw with which he has been sculpting the long-dead tree. We talk about his project through the blue veil of the scaffolding's netting, and I glimpse the outline of a totem pole looming behind him. Chainsaw, chisel or axe – Morganico's dad was a carpenter and trained him to work wood. I leave the artist to his carving and make a note to return for the unveiling.

The Chartist Tree, Kennington Park
Platanus × acerifolia/London plane

I amble clockwise around the park under the spongy arms of cork oaks that fringe the grass. Great groves of these trees, growing in southern Europe and North Africa, are stripped every decade before re-growing, providing the world with

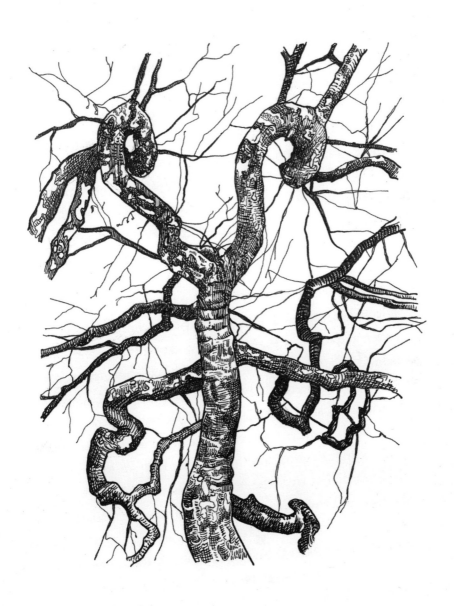

natural cork. I'm tempted to peel off a piece and take it home to be stored, then steam cleaned, before punching my very own bottle stopper from the bark.

High above the oaks a dirigible is revolving slowly over Kennington. The face of a smug dachshund stares down from three hundred feet, advertising who knows what and looking like it's about to defecate over Lambeth. The bored balloon crew chip golf balls around a cordoned-off area where the monster is tethered.

There's a funfair in full swing in the centre of the park but a group of children have abandoned the rides for a tree growing close beside the Tinworth Fountain. They climb in and out of branches that would break under my weight and, reluctantly, I walk on.

On the verge of exiting the park's southern end, and dejected at having not chanced upon a climbing tree, I pass under a spider's nest of branches sprawling over the fence onto Camberwell New Road. A London plane twists above me, the trunk's great S-bend yawning overhead. A wooden knuckle, eight feet off the ground, appears to be the only way into this majestic headpiece, so I call up a friend in Brixton and ask him to come and help me in. Half an hour later we are both poised over the road's busy intersection, kings for the day and each sitting on our own curling prong of the crown. After a happy afternoon watching the traffic, we take it in turns to make the awkward descent, and, as I slide back down the trunk, a huge cheer erupts from the Oval where a crowd is watching the final Ashes test. It's a fitting way of expressing my feelings for this muddled old tree.

The Magic Carpet, Normand Park
Cedrus deodara/Deodar

Next to the pool and health club in Fulham's Normand Park is a crooked cedar, stooping over the pathway. A branch with an upturned end, like the arm of a waiter holding a tray, beckons me towards the tree. The south side of the deodar is ringed with cider bottles – someone drowning their sorrows in the sun – and I tiptoe across these before clambering into the branches.

The climbing is heavy going in hot weather and I pause halfway up, resting on a huge crossbeam that extends towards the car park. Beneath my hands thousands of ants swarm up the deep orange rivulets in the bark. I lever myself higher up until I squat underneath the ceiling of the tree, shaded in a dark netherworld of needles. A group of men exit the gym and one of them breaks away, running under the tree and pissing against the trunk. I wish I could drop hard cones on his head, but this tree is still too young to have developed any – most cedars take at least forty years before their first crop.

With a final step up, my head and shoulders breach the canopy and I find myself in bright sunlight surrounded by a mass of swaying fronds. In its native mountains these pendant branches would be perfect for shedding snow. The topmost limbs fan out to form a level spread, and I lean back with no fear of falling through. To the south, tower blocks rise over Fulham and clouds dip low, scudding across the city's skyline. One of the ants tops out and takes in the view from my outstretched arm.

Normand House once stood on the site now occupied by the health club. It served as an asylum, then a school and briefly as a convent, but was finally torn down after being bomb damaged in the Blitz. Back on the ground I duck into the foyer of the gym and ask the receptionist if I can use the toilets. He looks at me coldly. 'Did you use the facilities today?' I think about the natural climbing frame on the doorstep but decide not to argue the point, crossing back over the road to a pub and leaving the cedar's roots unsullied.

The Guardian Tree, Crystal Palace Park
Quercus ilex/Holm oak

I alight from the train at Crystal Palace in hot sunshine. The tarmac path seems to bead with sweat as I cycle south, following the loop of the park perimeter. I stop in the shade of the concert platform, a slope of rust-red weathered steel. Across the path a copper beech stretches an enormous silver arm towards me. I spend five minutes vainly trying to reach for it while, nearby, a small boy is similarly engaged, clambering up a cherry tree that's no more than a sapling. It's hard not to envy a child's sense of scale, every climb a cliff face and every tree a giant.

Heading north through the park, I pedal up the border of the vanished palace past a fenced-off section behind mesh netting. The stone steps are cracking and a forlorn statue sits hidden in the shadows. Fencing has encouraged vandals, and

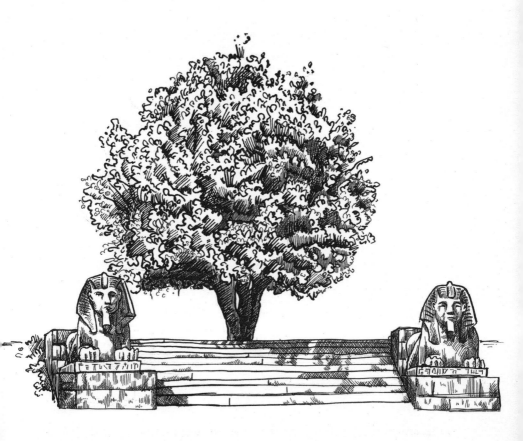

a plinth, covered in red and blue graffiti, features the 'Holmesdale Fanatics Ultras', the call sign of the local football fraternity.

On the Upper Terrace I stop under the hollow gaze of two sphinxes. Flanking the staircase that once formed the palace's north transept, they crouch implacable on their plinths. Victorian replicas of monsters from the reign of Amenemhat II, a pharaoh who lived nearly four thousand years ago, they have a hypnotic aura. This is heightened by the evergreen tree they now guard at the top of the stairs, a holm oak that spreads like a green torch, perfectly aligned between the sphinxes. Passing these gatekeepers, I feel I should go on bended knee.

A couple of ground-sprung branches have been pruned, and I step into the tree on their stubs, traversing in a circle a few feet off the park floor. This is a tree for reclining in, and I lean back on three wooden rungs. Gusts from all four corners of London lift the branches and my fingers rest on the bark's rough grain; it has the same pattern as a charred log, fragmented and cracked.

Behind me a tall hedge of spruce creates a solid wall, above which the BBC's transmission tower – broadcasting continuously since 1956 – rises seven hundred feet into the sky. The dull hum of the transmission unit seeps through the leaves. Looking back across the slope of the park, airborne thistledown drifts across the terrace and a swamp cypress floats like a balloon over the stadium lights, a still from a Miyazaki film.

The oak is a fine seat but a limited climbing tree, so I go in search of another ladder. At the east end of the terrace a hoary horse chestnut sprawls over the stairs, arms akimbo. Wasps swarm in its upper branches and I soon find the source, a large watermelon sculpted into a dragon, with toothpick fangs and a mouth full of insects. I climb down hastily, leaving the disturbing idol and its congregation behind.

The Corkscrew, Battersea Park
Platanus × acerifolia/London plane

In a quiet corner of Battersea Park lurks my favourite of all the city's plane trees, rooted on the bank of the boating lake. This is no light accolade, considering the capital is stuffed to capacity with these eponymous, tangled monsters.

A huge bole rises from the mud before splitting into two curling arms that fuse together in a central arch. Beyond and above, the tree becomes a rollercoaster, thick limbs spiralling in every direction. The jewel in the canopy is a high branch that curls over itself, forming a complete loop like a cowboy's bull whip.

The lowest reaches of the plane have been scrawled on by passers-by, keen to leave their mark, but these initials are flaking away as the plane sheds old scales. There is something reassuring about the tree casting off these would-be pretenders, short-lived animals trying to link their legacy to its own. One defaced branch swings low over a fake rock outcrop; the lake area is dotted with these strange cement boulders, as if the park visitor is trapped in the enclosure of a zoo.

Like all planes, the tree does not give up its secrets without a struggle. The wide bole offers one solid burr; I use this for hands and feet, stretching to plant my chest in the gap between the two branches. Turning to the western arm, I find a reassuring handhold in the saddle above my head and bridge the arch before pulling up into the crown.

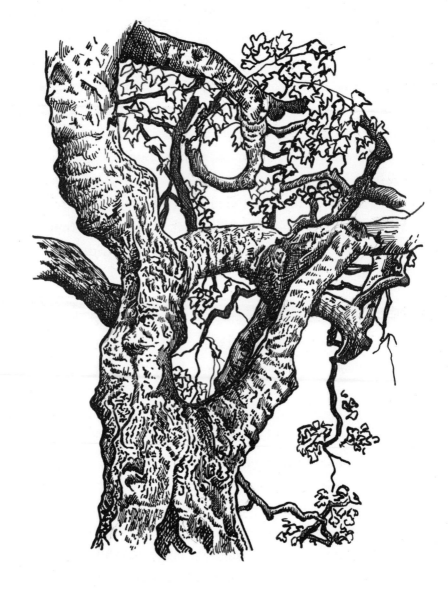

The high plateau that awaits the climber is like no other in London. Massive arms spread in three directions, kinked by the pollarding of long ago. The limbs have knobbly elbows, like old men with skin falling away from bone, and moss has gathered in the bark's creases. Another nest of jumbled branches crosses out over the water and I shuffle up an incline to crouch above the lake. Even though the platform is thicker than my waist, I move cautiously on the plane's smooth bark, twenty feet above the water. Standing up, I find myself level with the bull-whip branch and stick my head and shoulders through its centre, leaning on this magical loop in the sky.

Dropping back through the layers, I vow to return soon. When it dies this tree deserves its own obituary; a chronicle of how the centuries and the saw shaped its curling wings, and a lament for when it is no more.

The Strangled Oak, Battersea Park
Quercus cerris/Turkey oak

There are over a hundred species of tree in Battersea Park but the strangest of them all is a common oak. Standing next to the clapboard of the park fitness centre, the tree writhes upwards, its trunk ringed with curious scars. The bark is squeezed into ridge lines, puckered seams like the stitches of a fresh wound.

What warped the oak remains a mystery. Perhaps the trunk was wrapped around with a thick vine of honeysuckle and as the oak grew it expanded through the tight hoops of this parasitic vine. Equally, the moulding of these extraordinary contours might be the result of pruning gone awry or a mismatched graft.

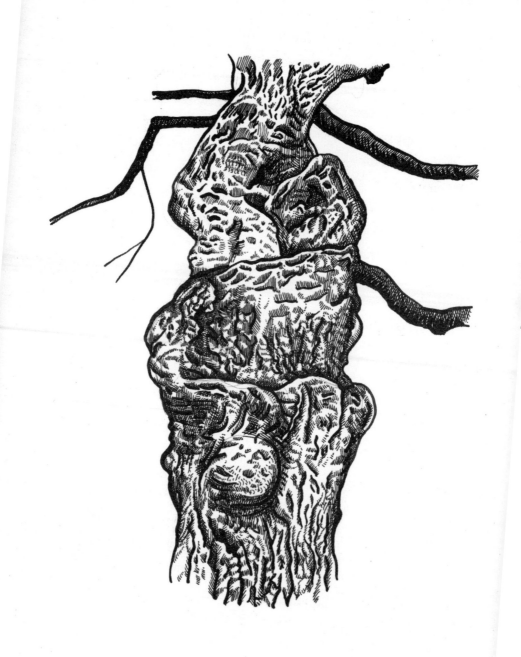

Whatever the cause, one happy consequence of the oak's disfigurement is that the branchless lower trunk has been rendered climbable. The rampart created by the scars provides a pathway for my ascent, snaking around the bole like the slide on a helter-skelter. I work my way up towards the crown by locking my hands on the outward-thrusting ledges and tiptoeing up the sloped rim.

I'm climbing on a damp day and feel unsure of my feet on the green wood as the ground recedes beneath me. At twenty feet the trunk's stairway gives out, just as the lowest branch of the oak draws within reach. A nervous hoist onto the south side and I leave the ridge line behind, trying not to give a thought to my return. Up in the canopy a view unfolds to the east of varied tree tops, with the iconic chimneys of Battersea Power Station behind. I sit on a high branch and watch gulls wheel across the park from the river.

The Totem Pole, Roundwood Park
Populus × canadensis/Hybrid black poplar

The road to Roundwood Park is paved with tombstones and I take a detour through Willesden Jewish Cemetery. I cycle down long rows of memorials, losing my way among marble epitaphs and finally breaking free under an avenue of horse chestnuts with a sign advising 'Beware of falling conkers'.

Entering the park, I walk past an oak clinging to the hill-side. Its trunk has a large open dial at head height, the remnant of an old limb, and a black memorial plaque has been hammered on to it commemorating Lance J. E. Hamilton. Long-dead flowers hang from a nail in the bark.

On the cap of the hill lies the bone-white body of a giant poplar. The tree's thirty-foot span offers a horizontal tight-rope, and as I approach a man is leading his daughter along its length.

This prone trunk might be the most tattooed deadwood in all London. The grain has been scratched across, scribbled on, hacked into and carved out with a thousand declarations of love: 'Priya loves Jai,' 'Buda loves David,' 'God loves us all.' On the north side a Latin inscription has been etched in six-inch letters: '*Te amabo in Aeternum*' – I will love you forever. Elsewhere, Arabic sits alongside Urdu in this great tablet of a tree.

At its eastern end the severed roots of the poplar still stand in the ground, the bark decorated like a totem pole with cryptic designs: diamonds and pyramids. Peering over the lip a hollow flute runs down into the soil, marking the rot that killed the tree.

Climbing onto the trunk, I join a small congregation already seated and gazing out toward Wembley Stadium's broad arch. I idle on the old log, watching as a race unfolds down the path, a crowd of competitive mothers and scream-ing children careering downhill in search of glory.

The Jigsaw Tree, Burgess Park
Salix × sepulcralis/White weeping willow

Owing to its haphazard assembly the greensward of Burgess Park is a jumble of relics. Unlike London's Victorian-era parks these Camberwell acres were not set aside but cut out of the existing city after the Second World War. Buildings were bulldozed and old roads rerouted, creating an uneven space. Walking the park's length, I pass iron bridges spanning long-drained canals and lime kilns squatting in empty fields.

I follow a random path and an ill wind fills my nostrils, a haze of weedkiller administered by a figure in *Ghostbuster* attire. He matches me step for step, hosing the ground as we go and suppressing nature in favour of a trim lawn.

On the bank of the park's pond, close by the Cobourg Road gate, is a magnificent willow. The tree is one enormous ripple from root to tip, with bark as liquid as the water behind it. The lowest limb unfurls within reach of my hand and I grab and release it, the branch springing back like the tail of an arrow striking home.

Groundsmen pass by with leaf blowers kicking up a storm at my feet. Without a piggy-back the first branch is a lofty goal and I crouch like a grasshopper before leaping for the topside. The tapering stem spans over the pond and I climb out on a promontory of willow wood. A mass of leaves shields the view but I can glimpse the white arms of poplars over on the north bank. Two men in iridescent business suits pass beneath my bough and look up with disgust at the naked soles of my feet. I watch with grim satisfaction as they attempt to wade through the geese that throng the waterside, their brogues soon smeared with guano.

Dropping out of the tree, I wander through a group of sycamores, one with a root cluster that acts as a stool. Over Trafalgar Avenue on a small patch of turf by the Surrey Canal Path another sycamore sprouts, with two stems flanking a central bole. I climb on branches that tusk at sharp angles to the trunk, pausing fifteen feet off the ground. The loops of an old swing cut into the branch, bark swollen over rope tassels like long-worn bracelets.

Species

Heart-halt and spirit-lame,
City-opprest,
Unto this wood I came
As to a nest.

'In a Wood', Thomas Hardy

The first tree I ever climbed was an apple that stood at the bottom of my parents' garden. I was five and it seemed enormous, indisputably the biggest tree in the world. I'd never heard of a giant sequoia, and if someone had shown me a picture of one it would have seemed like a shrub alongside that stupendous fruit tree. Climbing into the apple's branches took a leap of faith, but once aloft the world below became impossibly remote; my mother and father were dwarves, the family dog reduced to a hamster.

One afternoon I stole a chopping board from my mother's kitchen and wedged it high in the branches. It made a poor treehouse but I spent many hours squatting on that tiny lookout, transforming the lawn by turns into bottomless ocean or rolling desert. The ability of children to construct all-absorbing fantasies is amplified in tree tops – it's excellent headspace.

Years passed and new tenants moved into the tree in the form of a wasp colony. The apple is still alive but I cannot relate it to that giant of my childhood. It is just another unremarkable tree in a small orchard.

In London it is possible to find trees from all corners of the globe. By the reckoning of the Royal Horticultural Society there are over a thousand species rooted around Britain. Not every one of these grows inside the M25, but the spectrum of the city's trees is enormous, as is the diversity of their origins. Side by side with natives grow trees more used to high mountain or tropical swamp than London clay. While a few rarities are confined to the false light of greenhouses, many thrive in the open air. The city's trees are as cosmopolitan as the people who inhabit it.

How has our treescape evolved over the millennia? The trees we like to call 'native' have only been resident for a geologically insignificant period. Twelve thousand years ago barely a tree stood in Albion; much of our landmass was buried under an ice sheet and, with the possible exception of one very woolly variety of willow, little plant life of any size thrived at all. As soon as the ice began to retreat a great migration took place; seed by seed and tree by tree, beech, oak, ash and many others crossed the bridge of land that once connected us to the continent. In a window of a few thousand years Britain was re-colonised before rising sea levels turned her into an island. The pilgrims' route of our native trees now lies three hundred feet beneath the North Sea.

A total of thirty-four species are thought to have made this remarkable journey, though not all of these would have found London's marshland to their liking. Even so, it is fair to assume that a number of them have long been dwelling in the Thames Valley.

For several thousand years virgin forest, home to wild boar and wolves, stretched across most of Britain. Then, long after this Wildwood started to be cut down, beginning in the Neolithic, foreign trees arrived with foreign ships, invaders and conquerors bringing with them species now well established in British soil. Some of these were seeded by accident, others planted by the homesick as a reminder of far-off lands. A famous example is the sweet chestnut, a staple diet of the legionary and thought to have been introduced during the Roman occupation. Picture a soldier of long ago, exhausted and disorientated, dropping the first chestnut underfoot on the banks of an unfamiliar river.

Our more immediate 18th- and 19th-century predecessors were passionate cultivators. Empire builders were often compulsive collectors and brought home all manner of flora from their far-reaching travels; the tourists of yesteryear were likewise more interested in germinating rare seeds than collecting fridge magnets. Many of the great trees of the world were introduced to our streets and parks, from the cedar of Lebanon to the sequoia, and today these ornamental giants thrive in London, some proving better suited to city living than our native species. From nurseries around the capital these introductions soon spread across the gardens and parkland of the British Isles.

Whose were the hands that planted London's trees, fifty, a hundred or a thousand years ago? The descendants of these trees are all around us but it's easy to ignore those we live alongside. Next time you pass one in the street, pause and consider its ancestry. For an ancient oak, as few as twelve generations have passed since the thawing of the ice.

I am not a botanist. Neither am I a silvologist, dendrologist or taxonomist. Once, I dabbled in becoming a tree surgeon but was thwarted by an inability to wield chainsaws without consequence. I'm not even much of a gardener, as the troubled cacti on my windowsill attest, and if you pulled my knowledge of trees from the plant pot of my brain the roots would be shallow and the soil loose.

In the course of exploring London's canopy, curiosity has led me to bury myself in the deadwood of reference books. Even with these materials to hand the city's trees can be endlessly confusing in their permutations. The broad categories of coniferous, deciduous, softwood and hardwood present all kinds of difficulties, and it is easy for the novice to go astray. To further complicate things, urban trees are often pruned into bizarre shapes, sculpted to avoid traffic lights, bus shelters and rooflines, or to stop councils being sued for falling branches. From a distance these deformed crowns can be hard to place, their amputated branches contradicting natural growth. Many hybrid trees, cross-breeds of mixed parenting and cultivation, add another confounding element to the mix.

Sometimes I find myself circling the foot of a tree and muttering like a madman. I can spend hours staring cross-eyed into the foliage trying to identify leaf, bark or bud, but the cure, more often than not, is to climb into the tree itself. Here we can observe and absorb details invisible from the ground. A branch that you have held in your hand sticks in the memory longer than one seen from below. Squatting at the foot of a tree leafing through a handbook is no match for swinging around in the canopy. The more you climb, the more instinctive identifying trees becomes, the shapes of different species ingraining themselves in the climber's psyche.

What do we look for in a good climbing tree? Aside from a way up and down, there is no universal answer to this. There are different pleasures to be derived from the tree straight as an arrow and that which sprawls like a squid. Our anticipation on seeing a distant silhouette is heightened by never knowing quite what we'll find at the roots.

We look for different qualities in trees and, as with all things, we quickly develop favourites. Our ancestors might have sought shelter in one and firewood from another but today our preferences can be more arbitrary. I find myself drawn closer to some species than others, and there's an interweaving of a tree's characteristics with our own person-alities. Some of us might fancy ourselves the tallest tree in the wood, the first to feel the wind, proud and quick tempered in a storm. Others may be drawn to the well-shaded canopy and leaves that tickle the ground, or the indecisive tree, a tangle of branches spread in all directions.

Perhaps the most important trait in a climbing tree is complexity; the more it twists and turns, the more engaging the ascent. Tall ladders are always tempting, but height alone is not the marker of a great tree, and branches that can be explored from elbow to tip are the true grail. For all this, never overlook the merits of a simple perch – even a humble tree can make a fine escape.

Trees, like people, get more interesting with age. Their stories accrue and the wrinkles of time, in bark as in flesh, represent scars of growth and habit. Climb a veteran oak or horse chestnut, and centuries of experience can be traced in old wounds, the hanging burrs that stipple thick trunks offer a legible history of trials undergone. Passing under ancient boles, we are visitors at the bedside of the dying, a crop of green leaves like the twinkle in an old man's eye.

A great literature exists on all aspects of tree biology but the climbing merits of particular species are rarely, if ever, alluded to. What follows is an account of some personal favourites.

Broadleaves are this climber's first choice. Branching out irregularly from almost any given point, their climbing potential is infinite in its variety. Different species offer limbs solid as rock or supple as a springboard, while some canopies shift in the wind and others seem set in stone.

The most welcoming of all trees is the English oak (*Quercus robur*), which seems to stoop down and pluck the climber off the ground, extending long branches to offer a way up. What at first appears an unassailable trunk can often be reached by means of winding pathways from branch to bole. The arms of oaks offer reassuringly sturdy passage above ground – this is the same timber from which we have built generations of houses and ships. I never feel more secure than when perched in an oak and can happily dangle feet from high branches, unperturbed by creaking wood or the sheer drop below. Their great age gives oaks an aura of permanence and the spread of their crowns suggests a well-established order.

English oak is central to the English imagination, but many other species of oak grow across London and each offers something different to the climber. I have a special fondness for holm oak (*Quercus ilex*), one of the only evergreen trees to really thrive in the heart of the city. It provides respite all year round, a consolation in the dark afternoons of mid-winter when other trees are denuded. The bark is composed of hard-edged rectangles, providing good grip but liable to skin elbows and knees. A tree known by many names, sometimes the holly or evergreen oak, wherever it is found the climber will not be disappointed. The Turkey oak

(*Quercus cerris*) is another outsider that has flourished in London, growing to biblical proportions. There are fine examples in Ruskin and Dulwich parks, their thick limbs providing excellent bridges to journey up into the tree.

Oak plays such a central role in our history that the legend of some persists long after they are gone: the ghost of the Gospel Oak, a preachers' tree under whose branches the word of God was proclaimed, or the buried ancients of Windsor Park, vanished giants whose memory lingers.

A rival for the climber's affections is the horse chestnut (*Aesculus hippocastanum*). Introduced to Britain during the reign of Queen Elizabeth I, London is blessed with many grand specimens, their extraordinary growth patterns making them the most intricate of all climbing trees.

The bark of horse chestnuts becomes sharp and scaly with age, like the shells of molluscs, and provides a surface as pitted as the moon. The limbs of mature trees form crescents where they meet the bole, and there seems to be a warped endoskeleton beneath the bark, as if the branches cover innumerable backbones. Such is the extent of these hoary limbs, I sometimes feel trapped in a giant cobweb when exploring their spreading branches. In spring, horse chest-nuts produce the most decorative of all tree flowers, great pyramids of petals that hang around the climber like lanterns. Once pollinated, these transform into 'conquerors', the much-loved conkers that have bruised the knuckles of so many schoolchildren.

The beech is another broadleaf that makes regular appear-ances in these pages. The body builder of the woods, the thin skin of *Fagus sylvatica* seems to ripple with barely contained muscle. The bark is silver-grey and smooth, and, latched on to the trunk, a climber could be high on the granite cliffs of Yosemite. On bare sections the bark's even grain is intimidating, shrugging off the over-eager. But higher up firm branches twist and wrap around the trunk, providing jug-handle grips and rings of solid wood – excellent armbands for the novice. Beech bark is easily marked and heals slowly, and in the city you will come across tokens left by past climbers: initials, love hearts and cryptic drawings of every kind.

Beech was one of the last trees to colonise Britain after the thawing of the ice, trailing in the wake of oak and ash but forging forests all of its own – few other species being able to grow in the dense shade it casts. In the city the copper beech cultivar ('Purpurea') is hardier and more abundant than its parent tree; its purple outer leaf is an unmistakable homing beacon for the tree hunter. Never pass by a beech with a low branch; their upper reaches are whole kingdoms unto themselves.

Also much prized as a climbing tree is the ash (*Fraxinus excelsior*). Once seeded, it grows rapidly in favourable conditions, forming a graceful dome. When in leaf, ash provides a high, airy canopy, and sitting among its branches the climber could be floating on layers of cloud. It is a short season, however, and for those who relish the anonymity of thick foliage the ash is one of the last trees into leaf and the first to shed.

Mature ash trees develop deep fissures in their bark, allowing for alternative holds on branchless trunks. The branches themselves have excellent elasticity that lends a spring to the step of the climber. Ash wood is the handle of the world; its shock-absorbing heartwood has been used to craft tools for thousands of years and is as trustworthy a foothold as you could hope for.

Another abundant city tree, particularly along London's roadways, is the common lime (*Tilia* × *europaea*), instantly recognisable by its heart-shaped leaf. Common and large-leaved limes (*T. platyphyllos*) are tolerant of atmospheric pollution, as well as the aggressive pruning that street trees suffer. They are fast growing and reach lofty heights, twenty to thirty metres tall. Usually standing head and shoulders above their neighbours, they draw hopeful climbers to their feet only to be confounded by what they find.

Limes are the punks of the tree world, their growth all spikes and stray ends. These small shoots invariably make up the lower reaches, rendering the summit impenetrable. There's no tree that you're more likely to lose an eye climbing and, should you make it to the top, past pruning may deny you a comfy perch.

A final hazard is the sweet smell of lime blossom. Humans are not the only creatures intoxicated by the scent, and limes attract avid insect pollination. These trees are a favourite for bees and wasps, the climber's curse, and I have been stung by both in their branches.

More widespread in London than all of these broadleaves is the ubiquitous plane tree. The most common species is the hybrid, *Platanus* × *acerifolia*, a cross of oriental and American planes, commonly known as the London plane on account of its prolific planting across the capital. This plane is very hardy; resistant to pollution, disease and high wind, its roots are also comparatively shallow. On account of these merits, urban planting schemes of the past have favoured the tree, often to the exclusion of all others, and so it has taken over our city's highways and byways. The plane makes up over half of all trees in central London, and it is the most common border to our squares and roadsides.

For the climber, planes are the most frustrating of giants. The high crowns and their bird-nest tangle of branches make for glorious roosts, but the sheer trunks are daunting. The tree's natural urge to drop its lower limbs, and the council's chainsaw, ensure that few branches offer a way in. The flanks of older trees make for formidable rocky outcrops and the bark itself, shed and replenished every season, is prone to flake off under pressure. Many are the planes I have slid back down in painful defeat.

On this evidence it is tempting to ignore plane trees altogether and to despair of ever reaching their summits. But like all elusive arbours, those rare specimens that allow us into their branches reward with magnificent interiors. Coiled limbs follow eccentric paths, and the undersides of high arches are decorated with long lines of burrs, like the necks of giant reptiles. My favourite climbing tree in all London is, appropriately, a London plane, squatting on the banks of Battersea Park's boating lake.

In contrast to the spreading broadleaves, conifers tend to grow straight up and most are evergreen, providing cover for the climber all year round. Although these lofty green towers may at first seem forbidding, their branches are plentiful and often grow close together.

A well-appointed pine provides a natural ladder like no other, as if the tree evolved to be climbed. Each new ring of branches is evenly spaced as it matures. The growth pattern forms a dense spiral, and climbing a good specimen is as easy as ascending a staircase. The bark of most species is thick and scaly, providing reassuring traction for hands and feet, with smoother grip on the branches themselves.

In spite of the straightforward geography of their limbs, pines are messy trees to climb. I never emerge from their arms without a haystack for hair, thick with needles and pine resin. Thin, younger branches are also prone to snap and should be carefully avoided.

Britain's only native pine, the Scots pine (*Pinus sylvestris*), is a rare sight in the city. When full grown the tree's crown is often unreachable, forming a floating mushroom cap high above the ground. A lone example in this book is 'The Granny Pine' in Paddington Old Cemetery. A more practical species is the Monterey pine (*P. radiata*). A native of California and Mexico, it's now grown the world over both for ornament and its fast-growing timber. London is rich in these trees and they have provided me with some of the best aerial views in the city. In their crowns I find myself in splendid isolation, the ground invisible beneath thick layers of vivid green. Pines are long-lived trees and, where they're protected, should remain a feature of the cityscape for many years.

Competition for the best lookout posts in London comes from two species in the cypress family. One of these is a deciduous anomaly, the swamp cypress (*Taxodium distichum*), standing proud in shaggy majesty above London's treeline. Born on the banks of the great Mississippi, it was – and remains – popular with the city's waterside planters; nearly every park with a pond or lake has its own example. The species loves to hug the shore and in optimum conditions grows extraordinary 'knees' above ground, roots that aerate suckers permanently underwater. The champion specimens in this book are those close by St James's Park lake, tight-knit branches leading to ethereal domes. Their leaves darken over the course of the summer months and the canopy is best explored during their pale-green zenith in spring.

A second goliath is the giant sequoia (*Sequoiadendron giganteum*), an arboreal kingpin. Unlike the great citadel trees of the Sierra Nevada, whose trunks rise branchless for hundreds of feet, their London counterparts are easily accessible. Where they're found in park planting, enormous lower branches descend to the ground, protected against browsing and unthreatened by Californian forest fires. The tallest in these islands is probably in Blair Castle, Perthshire – measuring these specimens is an inexact science, and our figures are rarely for the current year – but a number of shorter trees are scattered across London's formal gardens. First imported as seeds in the mid-19th century, these trees are still in their infancy but can already transport the climber to great heights. Given space and the dignity to die a natural death, our sequoias will look down on us for many centuries to come.

Another conifer worth mentioning is the European yew (*Taxus baccata*). It is not an obvious choice for the climber, being a 'mortiferous' tree with highly toxic leaves, seeds and bark. A very small quantity of dried yew leaves is enough to kill a grown adult, say the amount of sugar you might sprinkle on your morning cereal, and their potency has led to the compound being adopted in modern medicine; yew clippings are used as an ingredient in taxol chemotherapy.

In spite of these drawbacks the yew possesses a compelling aura on account of its great age. Adept at propagating itself, branches touching the ground can root themselves to form new plants. Once a popular plantation tree, yew was the wood of choice for medieval longbows, the scourge of the French. The yew's cultivation goes back several millennia and the hoariest specimens in Britain are estimated to be over four thousand years old.

London has its fair share of ancients, and yews, unusually for a conifer, are tolerant of the city's cocktail of pollution. A short ascent will land the climber in their low, twisted crowns. Despite being categorised as a softwood, yew branches are denser than most hardwoods, providing ridge-like lines for climbing. The boughs of ancient yews are often rotten but also unusually thick for a tree of its stature. Sitting in their contorted limbs the climber feels like a time-traveller.

Of all the conifers the cedars are my favourites, and their climbing potential rivals the very best of beech and oak.

There are only four true cedar species, and three are common across the city: the deodar (occasionally known as the Himalayan cedar), the Atlas cedar and the cedar of Lebanon. As their names imply, all are mountain dwellers, their native ranges being many thousands of feet above sea level. Yet they have thrived at lower altitudes. Although they don't tolerate inner-city pollution, specimens on London's fringe are well worth the pilgrimage.

All cedars have an aromatic wood, and climbing through their branches offers a scented journey far removed from the city's all-pervading fumes. The oils in cedar wood were extracted by the ancient Egyptians, and the wood itself used to build thrones and ships. This makes cedars one of the world's first exploited species, and their natural ranges were being denuded many thousands of years before the advent of modern forestry.

The deodar (*Cedrus deodara*) offers an ascent closer to that of the pine tree, a vertical ladder with sprung branches. It is easily identified by its heavy, drooping foliage – you can remember this with the simple mnemonic 'D' of deodar, for branches 'descending' towards the ground. Exploring this thick drapery, the climber is completely enveloped.

The Atlas cedar (*C. atlantica*) and the cedar of Lebanon (*C. libani*) are an altogether different climbing challenge. Both trees have great plates of foliage, spreading up and out in successive strata. In *C. libani* these stacked tiers are perfectly level, leading to a flat-topped crown, but *C. atlantica* raises its arms and the topmost points skyward, the peak of a pyramid (hence the completion of the cedar mnemonic:

'A' of Atlas and 'L' of Lebanon for branches 'ascending' and 'level'). No other trees afford a comparable perch; broad, almost flat branches span celestial interiors. Caution should be exercised on very old cedars, as what look like enormous weight-bearing limbs can rot and drop without warning.

On those rare specimens where it is possible to climb unaided to the crown, the adventurer emerges on a plateau high above the city. The experience is as close to levitation as we can hope to achieve and the views are boundless. From the ground, passers-by will only see the feathered underside of the cedar's umbrella – the climber has escaped to another dimension.

People are astonished to learn that they can climb a giant sequoia or a tulip tree without leaving the bounds of their borough. In the chapters of this book are examples of these and many others; hornbeams and willows, alders and syca-mores, poplar, aspen and cherry. Explore widely. You will discover that no two journeys are the same and that every tree has a thousand eccentricities peculiar to its own growth.

Squares, Gardens & Greens

One of the city's great pacifiers – last bulwarks against madness and violence – are the garden squares and greens that cover it like patchwork. In summer these shaded dells offer a step down from the street; in winter a place of quiet meditation where every wristwatch loses an hour. These are the small corners of relief that all city dwellers crave and the calming effect they can have is quite remarkable.

Try watching harried commuters enter and exit city squares. The sour face that walks in through the gate is often a stark contrast to the one that departs – people stride in and stroll out. I once followed in step as a man in a three-piece suit crossed Brunswick Square. On entering he was visibly enraged, with a furrowed brow and clenched jaw. As his feet crossed from tarmac to grass, a remarkable transformation began to take place and his face softened perceptibly with every step. Passing into the shade of the trees his very gait changed, slackening in their shadow. When I overtook him exiting the far side that contorted look of a minute before was relaxed into a wide grin. No doubt if I'd trailed him on to the next busy street his former scowl would have reasserted itself. I wondered where his commute would carry him and if he'd pass through other greenery, his features in a constant cycle of emotion.

This chapter explores a wide assortment of city trees; those growing in grand garden squares and those guarding old village greens, now surrounded by buildings on all sides. Further afield lie gardens with age-old planting. Together, these spaces form a green artery and a soft interlude between bricks and mortar.

Sequestered in every corner of London, small gardens and squares are easy to pass by. We seek patterns in our lives and become accustomed to set paths, loath to deviate from an established way to and from. Of all the daily migrations taking place across the city, how many people pause to take in their surroundings? Your road to work might pass within a few feet of a climbing haven.

At street level these spaces exist inside clearly defined parameters, neat cordons that stake out their permitted limits. Look up, though, and they are overhung with the branches of trees encroaching on the city. Neat borders may stretch beneath them, but a tree is not a flower arrangement and will always fall out of place. The city's air space is unkempt and no set of iron railings can lend uniformity to the sky.

This untamed element in the midst of the carefully arranged is what makes climbing in these spaces so appealing. It is not always an easy task; gardens and squares are dominated by the London plane, of which only an occasional specimen can be conquered. In among them, however, there is always a stray branch to be found in the most unlikely of hidden corners. Finding and climbing one of these singular trees, we gain a lookout for observing the daily passage of city life. Forgotten objects are revealed to a bird's-eye view: odd statues buried in borders or the ghosts of old buildings and archways.

When every step on the pavement makes your joints ache and your lungs are black with exhaust, make for these small offcuts from the city's cloth. In their trees we can hide from the sensory assault of the street, the constant elbowing of crowds or the giant billboards whose eyes follow us wherever we go. Choose to step off the conveyor belt of the city, even for the briefest of moments, and you will discover tree-top retreats around every corner.

The Wooden Rose, Brunswick Square

Platanus × acerifolia/London plane

Rooted in the heart of Brunswick Square is a London plane that has been resident since the gardens were first laid out in the 18th century. Black, arched roots extend above the ground like hollowed-out sea caves supporting the barnacled bole, and two long arms unwind from above, old bridges crossed by many generations.

Moving to the south side the sun warms my back as I pull up on an elbow of wood decorated with illegible names. Ahead, the branch undulates like the ridgeline of a hill, the winter light picking out a speckled path into the crown. The bark is smooth, but small burrs freckle the surface and give the climber much-needed traction. I pause to admire one of these in the shape of a rose, curled layers of bark turned inward.

The branch is no more than ten feet off the grass, although the long ascent makes it feel very exposed. Reaching the trunk, I take a nervous step down onto the face of the tree with my right foot balanced on bark as slippery as pebbles in a river bed. Throwing my weight into the heart of the bole, I sway for an awful moment on the brink of falling forwards or backwards into nothing.

The risk is worth the reward and I follow the thick eastern arm high above the square, a grand perch from which to watch Bloomsbury. The square is never idle, its busy paths watched over by this tree for more than two hundred years. Below, three white poodles circle the canopy's enormous shadow, their owners conversing like well-heeled shepherds.

I leave the tree by a different route, sliding down onto the north flank, a dank and sunless realm where every wrinkle is furred with deep mould. On one side a large, rounded burr protrudes beneath a bird box, with a face and eyes like the carved boss of a cathedral choir. Reaching out to touch this strange effigy, I lose my footing, slipping sideways out of the tree and landing painfully, scattering pigeons to the four corners of the square. Looking up, I fancy the wooden face twists in mocking laughter.

The Black Horse, Temple Gardens
Aesculus hippocastanum/Horse chestnut

Beware! You're in a showboat garden now. Doing anything other than sitting sedately on a bench and sipping mineral water is deeply frowned upon. The gardens' by-laws, stapled to the guard rails, contain a wealth of zealous small print. To delve into these at random, it is forbidden to 'race or train a whippet', should you have happened to bring one with you. Singing is punishable by a fine, so if your chest is bursting to express musical joy find somewhere else.

Unsurprisingly, climbing trees is also prohibited. A fine of £20 can be levied on anyone caught up a tree by the garden authorities. When I was last there the garden authorities happened to be eating a sandwich on one of the benches – egg mayo, I believe.

Walking through the gardens, I cross beneath a statue of John Stuart Mill, a long-dead British philosopher who championed the freedom of the individual over the power of the state. Looking at John's expansive bronze forehead and curly locks, I picture him swinging from a tree in his tailcoat.

In the south-east corner of Temple Gardens there's a square wall of stone, tucked in among the shrubs. Behind it against the guard rails is a stately horse chestnut overlooking the Embankment and the river, and to get into it one must pass from wall to tree. Hoisting myself onto the parapet, I discover it's the cap of a giant underground exhaust, a void covered with wire grilles. Overhead the horse chestnut proffers a branch, reachable with a determined leap off the wall. Failure would result in a short but embarrassing fall into the garden shrubbery.

The branch is covered in soot, the combined fumes of the London Underground and the Embankment's four-lane traffic having turned the tree coal black. Climbing higher up, I gloat as a District Line service, containing several hundred sardines, rumbles beneath the rather roomy branches. I can feel the vibration of the steels through the tree's roots.

The little circle of garden benches looks quaint down below, contrasting with the giant granite façades of the Embankment's office blocks, ominous through the leaves. Over on the roadside, commuters tread thick and fast, every kind of hairdo and hat revealed to my airborne eyes. The horse chestnut is insect-pollinated and I watch nectar-filled bees being blown out across the road and the river, drunk from their feasting.

The Chrysalis, Fulham Palace Gardens
Sequoiadendron giganteum/Giant sequoia

On the lawn in front of Fulham Palace one tree scrapes the clouds, a giant silhouetted against the eastern yew hedge. The trunk is only glimpsed through a wall of green drapery, awl-shaped leaves extending to its base and brushing the grass. In the heart of the city a sequoia has seeded.

At first the foliage seems impenetrable but, circling the base, I come across an opening on the south side like a secret door. The branches part and I walk into a silent amphitheatre. When I look up, a spaghetti-armed monster looms among green cliffs, the tree's close-knit branches descending towards me as if squeezed through a sieve. The ascent seems daunting but the first limbs act like a springboard, bending almost imperceptibly under my weight and recoiling as I move higher. The lowest branches have an outer sheath of mottled pinks; growing alone, this sequoia will retain them for longer with no grove of older giants to overshadow it.

A few feet off the ground and the wall of leaves seems to heat the wind. I am cocooned inside the tree's veil and bathed in a warm, scented air – the fragrance of the American West. I could be lost on the tree's native slopes in the Sierra Nevada, with bears instead of tourists moving about below. Putting hand to trunk, the bark is orange and fibrous; a thick, fire-resistant skin.

I climb until the branches taper to twigs, taking care to move slowly and avoid breaking off smaller limbs. Stopping some way shy of the summit, I breathe hard, an arm around the soft trunk. To the east sixteen acres of allotments spread out on the far side of the yew hedge, an enormous patchwork of gardens. In among the jigsaw of greenhouses and scarecrows, and the long rows of root vegetables, small figures busy themselves turning the earth. Nearby, a spade flashes in the shade of a sweet chestnut. With a seven-year waiting list, these labourers tend their ground with pride.

Looking back at the palace, two other majestic trees rise through gaps in the giant's canopy. To the west, an Atlas cedar with stacked tiers of foliage spreading shadows across the lawn; to the south, down the line of the hedge, another American colossus: a coast redwood, shorter-lived than *Sequioadendron giganteum* but destined to grow higher.

On my way out I stop and talk to one of the purple-robed groundskeepers. She shows me the Georgian potting shed, with soil scattered across an uneven brick floor and a wooden

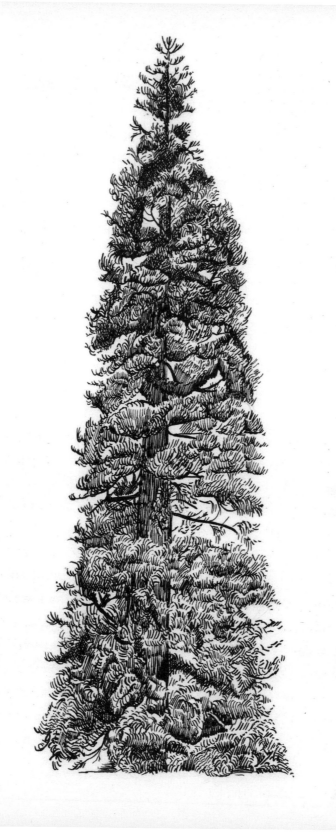

watermelon slice sitting in the window. The garden's tree survey reveals that the sequoia was planted some time between 1950 and 1971. It has a long way to go to match the elders of its tribe, well over two thousand years in age.

Bishop's Rest, Fulham Palace Gardens
Fagus sylvatica 'Purpurea'/*Copper beech*

The garden has slowly filled with children and some are trying to lift each other into the trees. Huge, sculpted pine cones lie on the lawn and the children roll over them or hide in their lee. A party sets up a picnic and, behind them, the copper mountain of a beech surges into the sky.

Stepping into the tree's dense shade, I find a man alone and lost in prayer, his hands moving along a string of rosary beads. Not wanting to disturb him, I step around to the far side before climbing up into the bole.

The waist-thick lower branches have patterns of concentric rings where they meet the trunk, piles of neat wrinkles flowing from the join. Higher up, I look back between my legs at the heart of the tree, a great arterial mesh of silver wood. The density of the leaves creates strata beneath me, cloud layers crossing the interior. They are dark green here, in contrast to the prized copper colouring of the outer canopy.

A view of the palace opens up to the north and the café spills out from its doorstep. People dutifully sip tea before going in search of the garden's landmarks: the ancient holm oak or the sculptures of dead bishops, hewn from the wood of a fallen cedar.

I sit awhile in a knot of branches, thumbing through a history of beech and its uses. The wood was once commonly employed for smoking herring, giving the fish a golden-brown colour and a much sought-after flavour. A long list of other beech-smoked foodstuffs follows, from cheese to beer, and a savage hunger drives me back down the tree.

Descending through the grey maze of the beech, I can make out children running in rings around its base, as if casting a spell. The branches encircle me as I drop through the layers, emerging from the dark understorey of the beech just as a group of young mothers passes by. They eye me suspiciously, as if I were the child-snatcher of a Brothers Grimm fairy tale.

I walk over to the walled gardens where a chiselled man is busy repairing the mortar on a Tudor arch. He gives me a precise chronology of every phase of brickwork on the wall and its Frankenstein history, before ushering me on with an impatient flick of his mortar board.

The Nostrils, Camberwell Green

Aesculus hippocastanum/Horse chestnut

Straddling the Church Street entrance to Camberwell Green is an old miser of a horse chestnut. Enormous flared nostrils greet me at the gate, the hollowed wounds from old amputations. Capping these great cavities, the perfect bridge of a nose rises into the crown.

I have to jostle my way through an army of pigeons fighting for food among the tree's roots. Walking around to the

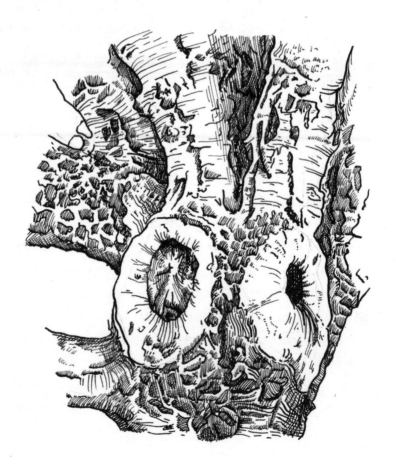

far side, I find that someone has deposited a large quantity of rich tea biscuits, a strange offering at the altar of the tree. The piles of biscuit break like a wave on the trunk but the pigeons seem more interested in contesting ownership of a lone waffle. Across the road a similar war is being waged at the buffet of Noodles City.

From the east side of the tree a couple of low burrs on the trunk can be used for footholds, enabling me to reach up and grab the U-bend in the branches above. An alternative way in is to grasp both nostrils, crimping my way left across the trunk until gaining the upper level.

The western arm of the tree thrusts out across the path towards the public toilets. Sitting on this, I am the gatekeeper of the green, confronting all who enter like the troll in *Three Billy Goats Gruff*. Around me hang the horse chestnut leaves, all badly browned from the caterpillar of the leaf-mining moth, which spends its summers munching through the foliage.

After I've been hanging out for half an hour a group of drunks congregate beneath the branch and start goading me, shouting, 'Jump! Jump! Jump!' Tempting as it is to throw conkers at them, I slip down the opposite side of the tree, crash landing in the pile of biscuits before making my escape.

Scurrying back across the green, I fall under the spell of a colossal London plane, bound and chained with electric lights. Black wiring covers the broad trunk and disappears seventy feet overhead. Continuing home, I daydream of using the lights like a cargo net to climb into this living lighthouse.

Pankhurst's Stave, Victoria Tower Gardens
Prunus avium/Wild cherry

Wading through lines of sentry boxes and camera-clad tourists, I come to a tall cherry tree guarding the east entrance to Victoria Tower Gardens.

Beneath the blossom is a memorial to Emmeline Pankhurst, her chiselled forehead rivalling a nearby Rodin reproduction. The frond of a weeping ash has been twisted through the statue's outstretched fingers, so that Pankhurst looks like she's enjoying a walk in the woods instead of battling the patriarchy.

I leap up to grasp a branch on the west face of the cherry. Great rolls of bark are flaking off at the base, the result of frost damage from past winters. A man in a grey suit, grey shirt and grey tie passes beneath, licking the ends of a roll-up cigarette. He gives me a cold stare – no doubt his eyes are also colourless.

Climbing the cherry, I find mature branches interspersed with rings of lesser shoots and am careful where I tread. The colourful bark is marked by horizontal bands, the easiest way to identify the species. This is a useful tree, with sweet-smelling firewood and fruit that makes a mean brandy.

Perched high up the trunk I watch policemen patrol the fringe of Parliament Square. Big Ben strikes the hour, five deep peals echoing out across Westminster. I can almost hear the collective sigh of the tourists milling below, another London experience ticked off the list.

The south-west tower of the Houses of Parliament rises through the branches, its sand-coloured stone and statuary stark against the blossom. Scaffolding runs along the length of the high gutter and tiny dayglo figures weave beneath Pugin's spires. The corridors of power are rendered invisible behind opaque windows.

Behind the cherry an easier perch is afforded by the low boughs of Elizabeth's English oak. Planted in 1977 to commemorate the twenty-fifth anniversary of the Queen's coronation, the oak has not thrived in its semi-circle of lawn but still makes for a fine retreat.

Exiting through the far side of the gardens I pass the cupcake of Charles Buxton's emancipation memorial fountain. This Gothic fantasy, with its fairy-tale crown, is a strange blend of materials, the red sandstone piers eroding fast under marble columns.

The Catapult, Lincoln's Inn Fields
Catalpa bignonioides/Indian bean tree

I skip across Lincoln's Inn to the strains of a cellist practising in the September sunshine. At noon on a weekday the park is full, and a devoted crowd gathers round as the musician switches from scales to Bach.

Nearby a fashion model is laid out on a picnic rug like a pale corpse, a camera crew adjusting the lighting around her. Above them stretches a far-reaching London plane, its mighty arms supported with rope slings and steel bolts, like a giant puppet waiting to dance across the lawn.

Wandering across the grass, I spy an Indian bean tree – there's a label attached to the trunk but the pendulous pods are a giveaway. It grows at an acute angle to the ground and, crawling up the sloping side, I squat in the fork like pea-shot in a catapult.

Owing to its ability to weather pollution, *Catalpa bignonioides* is a common tree across town, and a famous row of centurions flanks the Houses of Parliament. My own favourite grows above the grave of Stephen Holdrup in Wandsworth Cemetery and is worth a visit when its bell-shaped flowers erupt at the tail end of summer.

The Native American name for this tree is *kutuhlpa*, meaning 'head with wings'. Enormous leaves fan out above me, the sun illuminating their thick veins, and I imagine the roots being pulled from the ground and the tree taking off. An old woman in black and gold paisley pauses under my feet, putting her cigarette out on the trunk. She pockets the butt and moves on.

Circling the park on my way out, I talk to a shirtless man sitting in state on the memorial to Margaret MacDonald. His naked pot belly rivals those of the cherubim above and around him, as if he were an integral part of the sculpture. I exit the south-east corner of the Fields, past a hollowed-out plane tree with a hole in the trunk like the lip of a volcano. I ignore the temptation to climb it in favour of a pint in the Seven Stars, a nearby pub stalked by black cats in Elizabethan collars.

The Mountain Top,
Horniman Museum Gardens
Cedrus libani/Cedar of Lebanon

Frederick Horniman's stated mission was to 'bring the world to Forest Hill' with his eclectic museum and its artefacts from far-flung travels. I've come in the last hour before closing, but there are still crowds milling around the gardens and soaking up the view.

Many of the mature trees also represent distant lands. Not least of these is a cedar of Lebanon, standing on a high point in the gardens appropriate to its origins in the mountain ranges of the Middle East. It is one of the Horniman's most ornamental trees, most likely planted in the late 19th century when the old collector was still alive.

I heave my chest onto the lowest limb then scrabble with my arms and legs for purchase, doing a fine impression of the beached walrus in the museum next door. Once safely up, horizontal branches lead me to the back of the tree, away from the vigilant eyes of the gardeners in the nursery. The cedar's broad beams are easy to balance on as I climb higher until, twenty-five feet above the baked grass, the trunk splits and the broader stem leads to a gap in the terraced sea of needles.

The gardens are over three hundred feet above sea level and the view north across the Thames valley is spectacular. The skyline of central London shimmers between cedar fronds, the Shard rising like a modern-day Tower of Babel over a stack of lesser skyscrapers. I try taking panoramas

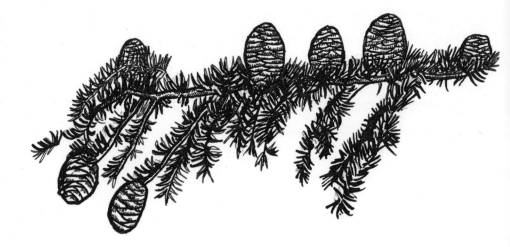

with my camera but give up, its lens unable to do justice to the all-encompassing scene.

The first notable cedars of Lebanon in Britain were raised in the Chelsea Physic Garden in the 17th century. Although these no longer exist, the tree was soon adopted as a crowning ornament of gardens nationwide.

Reluctantly I begin climbing down, a magpie chivvying me along. Near the bottom I pause by the stub of a pruned branch. The cedar's annual growth rings undulate like waves, forging a beautiful pattern in the heartwood.

Leaving the gardens, I pass an ancient oak propped on a wooden crutch and pre-dating the museum by a hundred or more years. According to the gardeners it would have marked an old field boundary, from a time when the whole of Forest Hill was farmland.

The Vanguard Beech, Lucas Gardens

Fagus sylvatica 'Purpurea'/*Copper beech*

A copper beech of biblical proportions, as wide as it is tall, confronts all those who dare enter Lucas Gardens. The tree's massive bole mushrooms above a path that splits to circle it, and there is no way in without paying your respects.

Some have done this with a knife – a malformed heart framing 'Reilly' and 'MYG' has left a deep scar on the belly of the beech. The bark has its own markings that meld with the old graffiti, swirling lines that garble lovers' names. At the tree's foot, water bleeds from the ground and I wonder if the beech takes its strength from a hidden spring, bubbling away under Peckham.

I sling arms around the lower of two eastern branches and hook my heel on its neighbour. Overhead the beech is an implacable granite cliff, and I struggle to reach the narrow V in the trunk and squeeze my body through, legs paddling the air like a terrier stuck down a rabbit hole. Squirming through on my chest, I arrive in a tangled wood; the knotted heart of the beech has a fairy-tale interior, a wickerwork of branches spun in all directions.

A wooden suspension bridge twists between the two main arms of the tree, off-shoots sprouting from its centre like steel cables. I worm my way up to it, nearly falling out at the far side; the drop is sheer, but everywhere I turn the tree offers wooden banisters to aid my passage.

Perched in the flat palm of the beech I peer down the north face. The stubs of lost limbs have formed into green ulcers

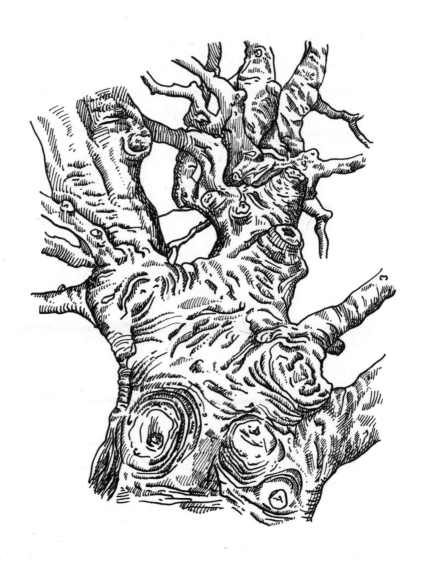

on the trunk, flat-topped volcanoes long since extinct. Elsewhere, radial patterns erupt at the joints of branch and bole.

At the south end of the park a man wearing oversized clothes attacks a blue guitar, addled hands no longer capable of a tune. Two kids on the neighbouring bench smoke a joint and speak in voices three octaves lower than puberty dealt them. On the boundary a square chimney rises over Vanguard Court. Now a series of artists' studios, the warehouse was once home to the Fibre Case Company (later Vanguard Luggage), a manufacturer that sent millions of suitcases out into the world until closing its doors in the 1980s. It's curious to imagine the survivors of this stock, still circling the planet's luggage carousels and carrier holds long after their bloodline has been severed.

The Amplifier, Canada Square
Acer pseudoplatanus/Sycamore

A constant hum fills the narrow corridors between tower blocks. Backlogged planes stack up overhead while giant air-conditioning units rumble at street level. Somewhere by the docks a pneumatic hammering adds to the cacophony.

In Canada Square a brass band desperately does battle with this sonic tide, watched by a small congregation of bored-looking office workers. Scrambling into a sycamore near the eastern end, I feel the enormous weight of the skyscrapers rising above me – they seem to lean in over the tree, threatening to topple.

A single figure hurries through the square. Nearly all life in Canary Wharf seems to be channelled over- or underground. Between the malls beneath the street and the towers overhead few people actually cross the open spaces. I'm reminded of Jonathan Raban's search for the Mississippi river in the heart of Minneapolis, a city composed of skyways and underground chambers. 'No wonder the streets had seemed so empty,' he writes. 'The city had gone somewhere else and cunningly hidden itself inside its own façade.'

A hopeful bird box or two has been nailed among neighbouring trees that fringe the square. If I'd migrated thousands of miles in search of a mate and ended up in this shit hole I'd commit the avian equivalent of *seppuku*.

On my way home from corporate claustrophobia I visit Jubilee Park, another green slice in the Docklands. A pall of smoke hangs over a fringe of swamp cypresses, the combined exhalation of a hundred office workers out on a cigarette break. In among them artificial pools lie undisturbed, and I wonder if the soles of sweaty traders find relief here in summer. The young cypresses will become excellent climbing trees a couple of decades down the line, but the park itself has the least friendly welcome in Greater London: 'The ways on this land have not been dedicated as highways, bridleways or footpaths, nor is there any intention to so dedicate them.' Ever.

The Gelding's Tree, Golden Square
Carpinus betulus 'Fastigiata'/*Fastigiate hornbeam*

Rounding the corner of John Street in spring, my spirits are lifted by the hornbeams of Golden Square ballooning out into the roadway.

A potted history is inscribed on a blackboard by the west entrance. Period drawings illustrate the square's sequence of ornamental layouts, from 17th-century box hedges to circular lawns and octagonal fencing. Underneath, the by-laws are twenty years out of date – be sure not to bring your 'radios or tape machines, they cause a nuisance'.

I climb into the hornbeam to the left of the entrance, taking a low perch nestled in its many-stemmed bole. The branches provide the security of a baby's stairgate, allowing me to recline and look up into the tree's spreading crown. The rounded canopy creates a perfect bubble above the square.

Circling to the street side of the tree, I thread my way higher, passing from outer to inner branches and back again. A step out onto a fork gives me a view across the square, with my heel balanced in the join. Hornbeam produces small but sturdy branches, giving rise to its nickname: 'ironwood'.

Directly below, the roots are invisible, covered by a protective layer of matting, a kind of fake wood-chip wraparound. The species thrives in London clay, and somewhere under the roots is the sealed-off cellar of an old air-raid shelter.

In the centre of the square, King George II poses in Roman guise, pigeons crapping in the folds of his toga. Arrayed in front of him like war trophies are the body parts of Josie Spencer's sculptures. The grisly torso of *Icarus Remains* provokes visions of a man tumbling into blue seas – if I fall from the hornbeam it will only result in a broken leg.

Hemmed in by Piccadilly and Regent Street, Golden Square is thick with human traffic and its small patch has been crossed by countless millions. It has morphed from political centre to wool market to media hub, but its finest residents are the hornbeams themselves.

Cemeteries
& Churchyards

The city is home to burial grounds of every denomination, order and age. Some have broad avenues behind polished gates, others weed-choked paths beyond listing fences. Many have vanished entirely under roads, railways and tower blocks; dead men and women whose remains lie sealed beneath our streets. There is not a corner of the city without its field of commemoration, whether it be a humble church-yard or one of the 'Magnificent Seven' garden cemeteries, enormous suburban plots created with the delusion that they could never be filled.

Disturb the ground under the city and you will soon strike bone; generations of cadavers have been interred in the substrata. Alongside recorded plots lie forgotten committals, the plague pits and hospital fields, the mass graves and private interments. In the 19th century London became so overburdened with bodies that the Necropolis Railway was founded, a funeral train running from Waterloo to Surrey with tickets for the dead in three classes of carriage, all over-seen by travelling priests. In 2015 Crossrail excavations beneath Liverpool Street unearthed the skeletons of three thousand mislaid Londoners, long trodden upon by daily commuters; everywhere we travel in the city our feet compact the faces of the dead.

This abundance of burial grounds has allowed trees to flourish, undisturbed for centuries in the heart of the city. The mature oaks and horse chestnuts, the grand old yews; all these have been thriving on human remains. Those bodies not encased in stone vaults or metal caskets provide sustenance for generations of growth, and even the most secure crypt is eventually seeded. Foolish souls who believed their bodies inviolate for eternity are now exposed to wind and rain, and roots carve channels through their graves. In this way, the city's dear departed have not left us but are mingled instead with the stems of our trees.

There is huge variety in the ecologies of churchyards and cemeteries, from overgrown jungles to well-ordered gardens, and botanical riches abound in both. Great trees grow in landscaped glades but also occupy neglected corners and unkempt graves.

Headstones themselves are often adorned with green motifs, symbols of rebirth and renewal: grapevines and lilies, thistles and oak leaves, poppies, snowdrops and sheafs of wheat – all these are carved into stone. The stone provides the substrate needed for lichen to thrive, hence the very grave markers themselves are patterned with new growth. Even the flowers that we leave for the departed, wreaths and garlands, find space to seed on the bodies of the dead.

The idea of climbing trees in such places may seem irreverent. Who would dare disturb the garden of rest? The examples that follow are, for the most part, confined to burial grounds no longer active or those converted to parks and playgrounds. Cemeteries and churchyards remain places of quiet contemplation, and I'd encourage all tree climbers to respect this; not to venture near graveside flowers or disturb those grieving or paying tribute.

But perhaps another form of tribute is to climb. If what endures of London's long dead is not tied to headstones but living in the trees, to climb these is its own form of eulogy. By climbing we observe the cycle of matter between the animal and vegetable worlds; the conversion of the dead man or woman to the living plant. What better way to honour the dead than to sit among them?

This transformation of corpse to copse is an idea expressed in Thomas Hardy's poetry. He sees the personalities of the deceased made manifest in the variety of graveyard trees:

So, they are not underground,
But as nerves and veins abound
In the growths of upper air,
And they feel the sun and rain,
And the energy again
That made them what they were.

The poet had first-hand experience of planting among the dead. In Old St Pancras Churchyard there is an ash that no tree lover should miss. Ringed at its foot, and entwined with its roots, are dozens of stacked headstones, moved there in the 1860s during the construction of the Midland Railway line. The new rails crossed an old burial ground, and Hardy, then working as an apprentice architect, was given the task of transplanting the bodies and their tombstones. The fine ash is a marker of their vegetable resurrection and its two-pronged crown shades the memory of many hundreds.

If you venture to climb the trees in this chapter, turn your thoughts to those buried beneath their branches. Do not assume that great trees are planted on great men – disappointment waits for those who seek only the celebrated dead. In Bunhill Fields on City Road the graves of John Bunyan and William Blake are overshadowed by stunted trees, and no broad canopies flourish above their bones. Sturdy trunks are as likely to thrive on little-known remains or unmarked graves. You may be climbing through the arms of a statesman or the crown of an undertaker.

The Three Crowns, Abney Park Cemetery
Aesculus hippocastanum/Horse chestnut

As I enter the cemetery the fattest rat I ever saw runs across the path, disappearing into the leaf litter. Its coat flashes ebony and for a moment I wonder if this is the true *Rattus rattus*, the old black rat of legend, hounded out of London by its larger brown cousin.

Abney Park would be a fitting last stronghold. An overgrown wooded wonderland, the tree-nesting black rat might be safer here than anywhere else. Once a flowering garden cemetery, Abney has had a difficult century and the grand old 'A–Z arboretum' has lost some of its former glory. But the trees have fared better than the cemetery's decaying chapel and, in among the undergrowth, some rare specimens survive: spotted thorns, unusual catalpas and strange-hued conifers.

From the entrance drive in the east I branch right three times until I find myself on the cemetery's northern boundary road. The horse chestnut's striking silhouette stands out on the footpath, three trunks with fenced crowns, like cupped hands raised to heaven. Directly in front of it is a tall stone memorial, mimicking the Egyptian revival style of the park gates. Here lie the mortal remains of William Hosford's wives, Amelia and Mary Ann. This is a family tree and I must ask permission before I climb.

To the left of the memorial stone the trunk has a large nook at chest height. Placing my hand in this cavity and balancing my feet on the bole beneath, I reach up for the first branch, trying to avoid using Mary Ann for leverage. The ascent to the first crown is short, ending in a five-fingered crow's nest fifteen feet off the ground. To the left are two further wooden strongholds, accessed by bridging the narrow gaps between them. Climb this tree with two friends and you each have a castle turret of your own.

Behind I can see over the cemetery wall into the upper storey of a glass building, Abney's wooded fringe turning the windows a subaqueous shade of green. Beneath the horse chestnut the graves of dissenters surround me. Founded as the first non-denominational garden cemetery, Abney attracted a menagerie of eccentric ministers and philosophers; the soil teems with men and women who refused to conform.

The Angel Pine, Brompton Cemetery
Pinus radiata/Monterey pine

Passing beneath the great arch of the northern gate I cross the threshold into thirty-nine acres of the dear departed. Brompton is a crowded cemetery, even with its vast catacombs. Everywhere you tread, coffins are stacked beneath you.

Pausing by the entrance, my eyes alight upon the cemetery's by-laws: 'Do not permit any animal of which you have charge to be tethered or graze.' I see a small pug tied to a gate, brazenly contravening the law, and take heart in my own quest to climb a tree 'without written permission'.

Branching to the left past the entrance, I follow the first path running south, a narrow corridor through the graves. In spring, waves of cow parsley break among the tombstones, marble crosses sinking in a sea of white. The path circles a roundabout of memorials and continues on the far side. Ahead stand two tall, flame-headed pines, their canopies floating seventy feet over the cemetery floor.

An angel presides underneath the eastern tree, serene in its shade and beckoning. You will know the pine by its long-buried congregation; a large snail creeps across the grave of Jonathan Glossop, wounded at Waterloo. I step off the path where the roots of the tree have begun to push through the tarmac beneath me, stretching to interlace with its companion on the other side. The pine has rungs aplenty for hands and feet, but to gain the first you need a helping shoulder or a bold leap.

Once among its branches, I climb through a network of upward-sloping beams. The sharp angles joining these to the trunk make for perfect handholds. The bark of the bole is deeply fissured, grey flecked with russet, but the branches are smoothed and green, the colour of bones long underground. As I gain height, patterns unfold in the headstones beneath: rows, circles and scattered mausolea. The white faces of the graves are stark against a foreground of bright-green pine needles. When the wind blows, the tree's fingers seem to be tickling the dead.

At the summit I sit among egg-shaped cones, holding fast to the spar-like top branches. A view for all seasons surrounds me. To the north, red-brick Victorian mansions rise over the tree tops; to the south, Stamford Bridge football stadium shadows the cemetery's central colonnade. Over two hundred thousand bodies lie in Brompton Cemetery, almost enough to fill the stadium five times over. Looking due west past the barrelled roof of the Earl's Court Exhibition Centre, I picture the many miles between London and the Californian coast, the pine's native clime. Descending, a blackbird alights on the branch above me, looking quizzically at a climber returning to his kin.

The Split Yew, All Saints Fulham
Taxus baccata/English yew

The churchyard at All Saints Fulham is sunk below the level of the Putney Bridge Road. Leaving bumper-to-bumper traffic behind, I follow an avenue of pollarded limes to the church door. As I arrive it begins to rain. Church wardens hurry past me, loaded with armfuls of pink and white flowers.

To the right of the lime avenue a gorgon's head of twisting limbs hangs over the churchyard, the tangled branches of an ancient yew. Standing under the tree, I see a split running through the trunk at head height and wedge a hand in this narrow canyon, thick cobwebs greeting my fingers.

Pulling up into the yew, I find a warped interior world of red-hued wood. There's no comfortable perch, so I squat between branches and survey the graveyard below. William Powell's Gothic almshouses march along the boundary wall, home to twelve widows, and beneath my feet illegible gravestones spot with rain. A litter of yew leaves, turned golden in death, covers the ground around them like a fortune cast aside. To the north lie three companion yews with contrastingly straight trunks; behind them a sycamore erupts from between stone coffins.

Taxus baccata has venerable ties to Britain's graveyards. Among the longest lived of all tree species, there are specimens in London over two thousand years old, relics from a time when the city was nothing more than a bunch of huts beside a river. Yew wood outlives even iron.

In spite of its longevity, the yew is as valued for its associations with death. Almost every part of the tree is highly toxic, and pastors of yore installed them in churchyards to keep grazing cattle at bay. No cows threaten to trample All Saints today but the tree remains highly poisonous; if I ingested a fistful of the dried leaves I would join the ranks of cadavers feeding the yew's roots. I look at the stains covering my hands and hold them up to the rain.

Back on holy ground I visit the church, where blue roof rafters support the ceiling and golden angels hover over the choir. Near the entrance a knight's chain-mailed gloves are carved in stone, the cast-offs of a long-dead constable. I fall asleep in a pew made from pine wood, listening to the rain lashing against the glass.

John Joshua's Lime, Hammersmith Old

Tilia × europaea/Common lime

Hammersmith Old is an everyman cemetery. Before opening in 1869 the land was the site of an orchard and a market garden, and something of the communal feel of both persists today.

In the centre of the cemetery, on the north side of the main avenue, stands a single lime. Visit in spring and summer, and you can climb unseen by the commuters in the tree's conical shadow, its heavy foliage drooping to within a foot of the long grass.

In season, buttercups and bluebells are found in equal abundance at the tree's foot, and men born many thousands of miles away lie buried among them. John Joshua, 'who fell asleep' in the year 1897, was a resident of Antigua, and close

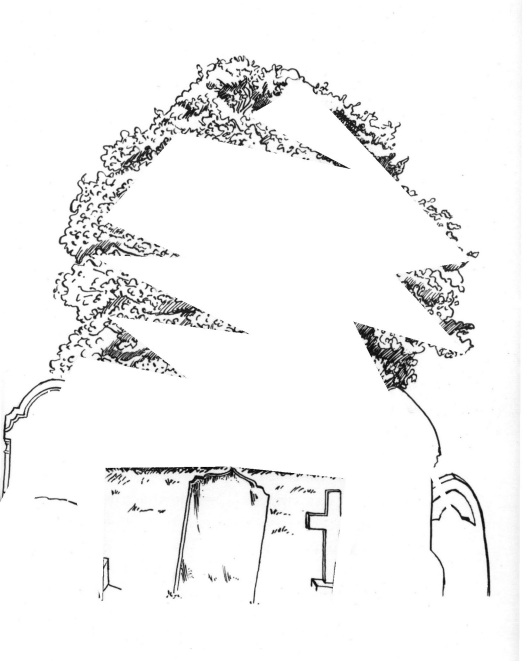

by his side is William Tracy, born in Kings Mountain, North Carolina.

The far side of the tree presents easy climbing to a fork twenty feet above the ground. As I ascend, glimpses of the cemetery's main thoroughfare show through the leaves. Crisp heels stride purposefully through, with no time to spare; more leisurely types sit reading books or eating sandwiches between the tombstones.

This is a tree for contemplation. The fork is enveloped by the lime's heart-shaped leaves, the city outside eclipsed by green curtains. I could happily while away an hour or more in total seclusion, but my own peace is broken by a wasp with sociopathic tendencies. It stings me on the forearm before buzzing off across the cemetery. The insult is quickly forgotten once I descend the tree and return to the main avenue, in part because I discover the grave of Sextus Gisbert Van Os. This wonderful character has his name inscribed on an opulent stone pillow, questionable cushioning for the afterlife.

If limes aren't your tree of choice, there's a squirrel-infested horse chestnut across the avenue, overlooking the screen-wall war memorial. Nimble climbers can also attempt one of the London planes in the south-west of the cemetery to get a peek at Queen's Tennis Club. Perch there on a sunny day in June and you might catch a glimpse of some of the world's tennis stars. You might equally catch the eye of the club's security and be hauled down to eat strawberries while awaiting transfer to Hammersmith & Fulham police station.

As I circle the cemetery on my way out, I find a cyclist pissing in a shaded corner of the memorial chapel. I stand looking solemn by the adjacent grave of John Wright to make him feel bad.

The False Prophet, St John's Wood Church Grounds
Acer platanoides/Norway maple

Entering the old churchyard, I find the gravestones occupying the fringe, as if some great geological upheaval has cast them from centre stage, now occupied by a clutch of picnic tables. Above one of these a maple with upswept limbs stands sentry and a man in a suit sits on the bench, his orange tie perfectly matching the autumnal leaves.

The tree is thin-armed, and I plot my way up before leaping for the first branch. The north side has been heavily pruned, forcing me to stick doggedly to a narrow climbing corridor. Where the wounds have healed, the underlayer is a deep chocolate brown, contrasting with the bright-yellow lichen adorning the upper branches.

As I climb a squirrel drops a shower of peanut shells from above. Confused, I soon spot the source; a man in a racing-green wheelchair feeds a host of scavengers in a corner of the grounds. He soon tires of his flock and moves away at speed, tearing across a kids' game of football.

The maple's summit has two saddle seats one above the other. Unable to resist the lure of the highest I wedge an

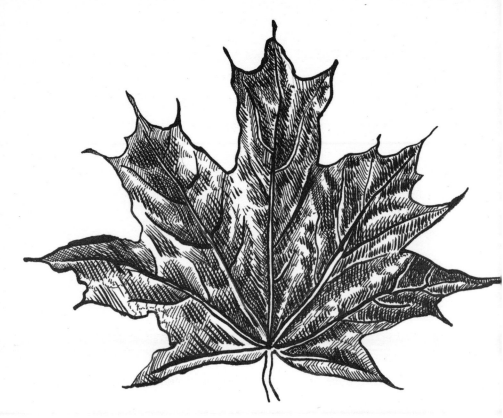

elbow in the crook, letting my legs dangle out over the church grounds. Palmate leaves cluster in great conspirators' circles, each similar in shape to the Canadian flag's emblem. A branch below my feet has an open canker deforming the bark.

The picnic tables fan out underneath, now closely guarded by two teenagers in baseball caps arguing heatedly with one another. Their conversation is borne up by the breeze:

Short kid: 'I'm half-Iraqi from my mum's side.'

Tall kid: 'You wish, bruv. She's from Yorkshire.'

I climb down, briefly interrupting the debate, then cross to the maple's immediate neighbour, a fenced-off tree with ground-hugging limbs.

Before leaving St John's I read a couple of the headstones, searching unsuccessfully for the infamous Joanna Southcott, a woman who predicted she would give birth to the second messiah on 19 October 1814. No child appeared, and Joanna died in December of the same year. Her followers refused to bury her until her corpse began to rot, fervently convinced that she would be raised from the dead. She now lies somewhere beneath the maple's shadow.

The Old Crutch, Kensal Green Cemetery

Carpinus betulus/Common hornbeam

Walking up the Harrow Road to the main gates of Kensal Green Cemetery, I pass the dusty shop window of E M LANDER, *Monumental Masons*. In a literal frame of mind I picture giant men with six-foot chisels carving the gravestones of dead titans.

I pass through the middle arch into the cemetery and am met by an old man with a wild white beard, a bona fide soothsayer. He sits mumbling on a bench at the entrance where I loiter, not knowing which path to follow. His eyes keep wandering to the left, as if searching for enlightenment there, so I take the track that twists away in the same direction.

Just before the cemetery's Victorian colonnade, capped with modern flats and air-conditioning units, I fall under the spell of an old hornbeam at a junction in the cemetery paths.

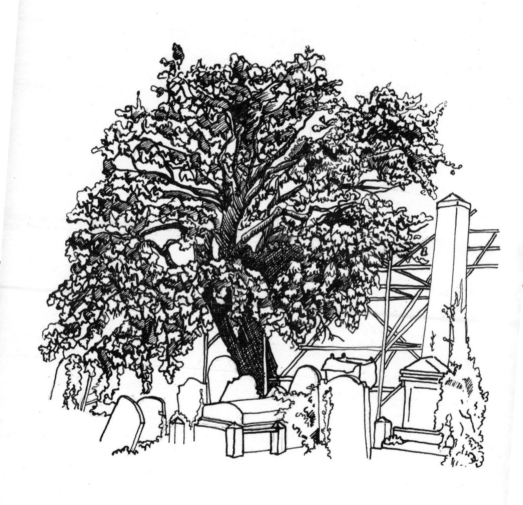

The trunk is almost translucent, with scored white veins threading the bark and the crown bending forward to overshadow me.

I use the scaffolding against the cemetery wall to climb into the tree. The prop is a reminder of the enormous cost of keeping memories alive; the maintenance of the garden cemetery must be a colossal task. As I cross from scaffolding to branch I read the graves of those entangled with both. Earl Minto Alleyne keeps company with Frederick Dewing; on the former's headstone is a verse that lingers in my mind:

Man covets heaven – but O that steep ascent,
How few in youth have stedfastness to climb.
Earth's happiest pilgrim would be well content
To gain that height, without the toils of time.

I sit in a cluster of branches, a low perch for reflection in this forgotten corner of the city. Motorbikes scissor the air behind the wall barely ten feet from my head, seeming to ride straight through the graves like the apparitions of England's last Hells Angels. In a lull in the traffic I flinch at a movement beneath the tree. A Doritos packet sails down the row of headstones, alighting at the base of an obelisk, a token of the world outside wafted over the boundary walls.

To the west the giant metal frame of a gas tower hovers on the horizon, pierced by the lines of Lombardy poplars marching along the cemetery's central avenues. Elsewhere, the disjointed head of Trellick Tower looms larger still, rising through a stand of horse chestnuts.

On my way out I pass a row of black Beamers with smoked window glass surrounded by a group of suited men in matching sunglasses, even though the day is overcast. One has a long scar running diagonally down his cheek and watches me as I go. Beside the path lies an ornate memorial, gold lettering on black granite. It reads, 'This Mausoleum is for demonstration purposes only. For prices, contact the cemetery office.'

The Black Hand, Nunhead Cemetery
Quercus ilex/Holm oak

The air is close and the light fuses vegetation into a solid wall, as if the whole cemetery were enclosed in a giant glasshouse. Tall spindles on either side of the path are unidentifiable as trees, buried alive by rampant ivy. It's hard to draw breath in this dense jungle of sycamore and elder.

The holm oak hangs over the path on the cemetery's eastern boundary, black fingers arched over the through road. I half expect to see a cloaked figure crouched on the bough, ready to drop silently onto passers-by. Instead, three little girls in pink and yellow play in the branches, their bright clothes stark against the graveyard's pervasive grey. Their mother draws on a cigarette, her smoke ringing the headstones and seeping into the undergrowth.

Once they've moved on I explore the tree. The oak lies horizontal on the ground, its trunk prone and the bottom branch eaten away, already sinking into the cemetery floor.

Crushed beneath it is a single cloaked urn, a broken symbol of immortality. I climb astride the trunk and then crawl up the arm. The perch is no more than ten feet off the ground and I sit in a gap between branches, like the two ropes of a swing in an underworld playground.

I follow the line of the tree back to its roots, where the bark is wrapped in thick moss. The base of the oak is obscured by a mass of ivy, and I walk through spiders' webs and chunks of broken stone in the leaf litter. I stub my toe on a half-buried headstone and fancy I hear underground laughter shake loose the soil. Peering behind the ivy cover, I find the tree's roots are half out of the ground. A fox has made a diabolical den in the gap between stem and coffin.

The name on one headstone is illegible but capped with an unusual design. The cracked spring of a carriage has been carved in raised relief and, above this, an epitaph reads, 'The spring of life is broken.' Whether this is the resting place of a coach salesman I will never know, but it fills me with dread.

Leaving the cemetery I pass the neat order of new graves, spared from the ivy. How long before they too are sucked into the undergrowth? I see the three girls again, now eating blackberries among the memorials, fruit that has grown fat on the dead.

The Granny Pine,
Paddington Old Cemetery
Pinus sylvestris/Scots pine

I enter Paddington Old Cemetery with a weak sun trying to colour Kilburn through a veil of fog. A path in the shape of a horseshoe runs alongside the perimeter and I cut across it to the cemetery chapel.

Steel fences ring the building's walls and yellow signs warn against falling masonry. I stare up at ornate chimneys vanishing in the fog and carved faces staring back at me from the eaves. A postcard attached to an information board advertises 'Tombstone honey' from the local apiary.

I turn due north up the main avenue and the sun finally dispels the shroud of mist. The first tree to emerge is a Scots pine, living up to its reputation as a landmark tree once planted to guide drovers home. Closer up, a second pine squats on the east side of the path, a low dome spreading over the ground. This is the bent back of a 'granny pine', a survivor from the cemetery's inception in 1855.

Pinus sylvestris, Britain's only native pine, is a rare find for the urban climber. North-west London is a long way from the tree's stronghold in the Scottish Highlands, where remnants of the Ancient Forest of Caledon form a nine-thousand-year link with the past.

Touching the pine's bark, the pattern is familiar to me – a hide of orange-pink scales that look like small thumbprints in the wood. The trunk slopes away at a forty-degree angle, wrapped around in thick ivy with horizontal limbs

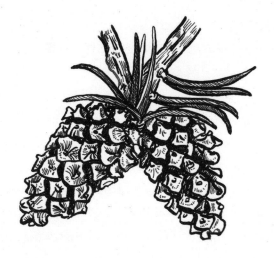

outstretched to the south. The lower branch swoops to the ground and curls back on itself, creating a ring-fenced den. I climb into this netherworld, sitting down only to leap to my feet again, the spiked leaf of a holly protruding from the seat of my jeans.

Behind me a line of stone vaults lies in the pine's shadow, their occupants' names obscured by fallen needles. I clear this bronze carpet from the first, revealing the tomb of one Elizabeth Prideaux. Across the avenue is a neatly trimmed memorial of the same age, a new headstone adorning the grave of Cuthbert Ottaway, England's first ever football captain.

Throwing a leg over the first branch, I move higher onto the parallel second storey and perch under the tree's tangled roof. The canopy overhangs my head and short branches grow into one another, with songbirds darting through long tunnels of twigs. Below, a father and son speed by on bicycles chanting the chorus to 'We Will Rock You'.

The Pulpit,
St Paul's Cathedral Churchyard
Liquidambar styraciflua/Sweet gum

I arrive at seven o'clock on a Sunday morning, an hour before Holy Communion. Cheapside is deserted and beer cans rattle around in the cold November wind. Crossing to the south side of the churchyard, I find a sweet gum in seasonal attire.

Liquidambar styraciflua is the crimson king of autumn, and the tree rises in the join between choir and transept, its foliage stark against the stone walls. Nearby a woman sips coffee in the shadow of an aspen. The benches below the sweet gum have been bombed by pigeons and their painted boards fail to tempt passers-by.

Cautiously, I step over a small fence guarding a flower border and start to climb the north side of the tree. Crawling up a steep incline to a lone branch, I swing around to the southern face. The scale of the cathedral wall is terrifying, and ascending the tree feels like climbing the mast of a sailing boat in the lee of a giant container ship. After a desperate scrabble, the cathedral dome appears through a blood-red ceiling of leaves.

In spite of numerous branches higher up, my heart is pumping as if gripped by a fever – I have never been more terrified or determined. I look down at the churchyard, where a splayed sculpture of Thomas Becket lies prostrate on the lawn, arms raised in defence. The head of the statue is thrown back, open mouthed, more like the cry of a man

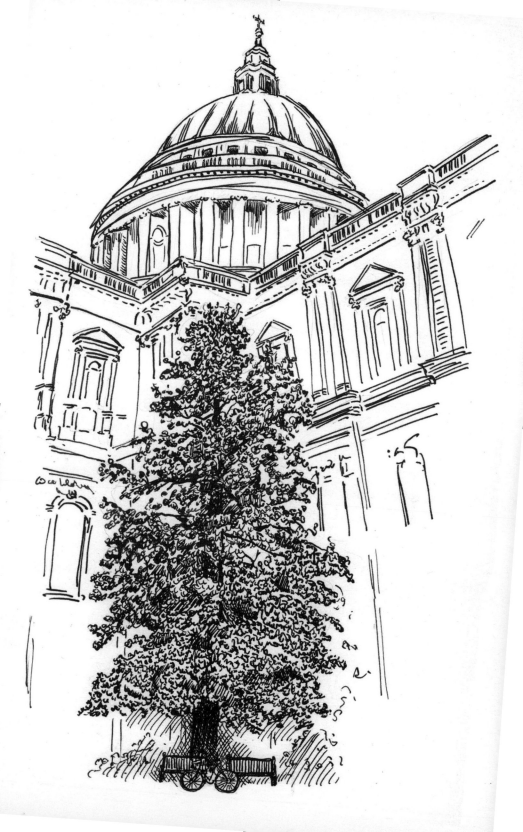

falling to his death than the face of a martyr at the altar. My fingers tighten around the trunk and my nails dig deep into the bark. No one would beatify a man for falling from a tree.

Overhead the great cathedral bells begin to chime the morning call to prayer. In my current state the sound is like a death knell and John Donne's famous words fill my agitated mind: 'Never send to know for whom the bell tolls; it tolls for thee.' The poet's own memorial lies a stone's throw away within the cathedral's nave.

I inch higher, and these fearful thoughts are banished on drawing level with the giant face of a cherub, a carving fixed to the cathedral wall. Roofline statues may be imposing viewed from the ground, but up here the angelic child wears a stupefied expression.

I dare not test divine patience or my own human strength by climbing to the zenith, and begin a long retreat the way I have come, trying to glimpse worshippers through the amber glass windows of the east end.

Back on the first branch I hang like a grape, dangling with the intent to jump down – what little I can see over my compressed chin seems impossibly far away. Finally, exhaustion forces me to abandon myself to fate. I drop with a hollow thud onto holy ground.

Royal Parks

We have a long line of dead kings and queens to thank for the existence of the Royal Parks, their common obsession with hunting leading to the enclosure of great tracts of the formative city. Through buying and fencing land for their own pleasure, past monarchs unwittingly preserved these spaces for the public, preventing them from becoming a composite of crowded streets. Today the odd regal ceremony still takes place, cannon salutes and fireworks, but for the majority of the year these parks are places of solitude and retreat.

When these vast areas were first cordoned off, who could have guessed how the metropolis would expand around them? What were once open fields on the city's margins are now vital breathing spaces in its midst. A green corridor threads through central London, from St James's to Green Park and on to Hyde Park and Kensington Gardens. Further afield, Richmond and Greenwich offer secluded glades to explore at will.

It is easy to be convinced that the Royal Parks have always looked just so, pathways and flower borders locked in stasis, unchanged for centuries. In reality, the whims of successive monarchs and the contrasting visions of landscape designers have altered layouts and uprooted trees. Some veterans have stood the test of time, but the parks have seen many periods of arboreal upheaval. The two world wars in particular took a heavy toll, many trees cut down for their timber or cleared to provide room for anti-aircraft guns and radar. Trenches were dug and space appropriated – the lake that feeds the swamp cypresses' roots in St James's Park was drained during the First World War, its dry bed used to build new war offices, the bridge passing over a canteen and a warren of bureaucratic housing. The picture-postcard view of Buckingham Palace was not always thus.

The Royal Parks chart the history of London's planting, and their many acres – balancing the scales and enabling nature to thrive surrounded by ring roads – should be cherished. Over thirty-seven million people pass through the parks every year, but how many pause to climb a tree? There is virgin territory here, unvisited perches that provide hide-aways in the heart of the city.

The parks are meticulously maintained and their trees trimmed to a fault, like toy dogs in a grooming parlour, so there is rarely a branch out of place. Many mature specimens exhibit scars at the bases of tall trunks, ghosts of former limbs and the paths a climber might once have taken.

In spite of this, there is plenty of opportunity to climb. The parks contain some of London's grandest and oldest planting schemes, and the most exotic species. Their open acres dominate both centre and fringe, from Hyde Park's green cavity to Richmond's rolling fields. Combined, they stretch to an area of nearly eight square miles and contain an estimated one hundred and seventy thousand trees. Whole days can be lost exploring the length and breadth of these arboreal riches.

Buried in the Royal Parks' by-laws is the admonishment, 'No person shall, without reasonable excuse, climb any tree.' Ambiguity is a glorious thing and the space afforded by the parks is great enough that the considerate climber can go about their adventures unnoticed, passing through the canopy like a human chameleon.

There are some notable absences here from the Royal deck; I have not ventured into the distant canopy of Bushy Park, and Green Park does not make an appearance until after dark, in the penultimate chapter of this book. Brompton Cemetery is also Crown land, but its climbing pine can be found in the Cemeteries & Churchyards chapter.

The Hermit Hole, Hyde Park

Zelkova carpinifolia/Caucasian elm

Scurrying across the intersections of Hyde Park Corner, dodging the occasional stray horse and cyclists who think they're in the Tour de France, I enter the park's three-hundred-and-fifty-acre hinterland.

Before crossing into the open fields at the heart of the park, I have to negotiate the formal gardens. These flowering lanes are preyed upon by pretzel vans and mobs of sightseers, en route between the city's main attractions.

In the thick of all this human traffic there grows a rare tree. It seems so alien to its immediate surroundings that people pause beneath it and peer with curiosity at the label pinned to its trunk. *Zelkova* – the name itself is redolent of far-off lands.

The tree is best climbed in winter when its colourful bark and striking geometry are exposed, branches thrust vertically like static hair. The trunk grows to a moderate height before splitting into a tight-knit fence of branches, and I jump to grab one of the outliers. A man leans against the tree, oblivious to my intent, his eyes closed and the chorus to 'Sweet Child of Mine' leaking from his headphones.

There's no way of falling out of the tree once in it, and I cross the wooden palisade into a strange nether realm. A second layer of branches creates a tunnel effect and, emerging into the centre, I feel as if I've burrowed in. All around me rise grey pillars with flaking scales revealing bright orange spots. Being lost in these branches is akin to being buried in a root system. I imagine myself a mole, twitching in the half-light that filters down into this wooden hall carpeted with leaf mould.

Occasional glimpses of Knightsbridge tower blocks intrude on the sanctity of the cave, but this is a tree for looking inward, not out. Recent pruning has left footholds that help me scale the vertical stems, and I gain a warped view back into the bole.

The Caucasian elm, much like the square-jawed men living in the mountains of the same name, is hardier than its English cousins, trees much mourned by those that remember

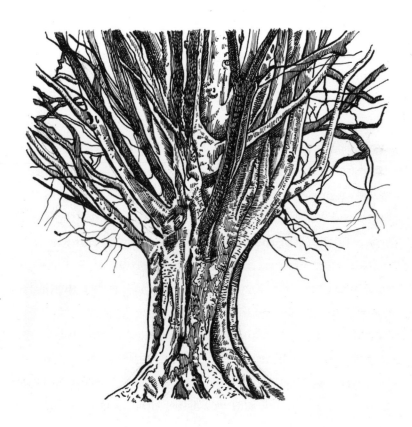

them. It tolerates the disease that wiped them from our landscape and killed three-quarters of those in North America.

Threading my way back out of the labyrinth takes time. Dropping out of the tree I find that gas lamps have flickered into life across the park.

The Pedestal, Kensington Gardens
Fagus sylvatica/Common beech

Set back in the open lawn behind Princess Diana's Memorial Avenue is a fine beech, the top sides of its branches green with mould. I stand in its shadow and the tree points a finger due north, from which direction a freezing wind blows, chilling my marrow.

I lever myself onto this outstretched limb, with my breath making thick clouds in the air. Directly overhead, a parallel branch leads back towards the bole, two smooth wires drawing me up into the tree. The bark of the trunk is a vivid bottle green, and I hook my arms over higher branches, hoisting my knees up onto the next level. Swaying forward in this position, I am prostrate like a priest before an altar. Beneath me, a neat circle of black manure rings the tree and the limbs appear like cut-outs against the soil.

Poised in the tree top, my view of the Albert Memorial is bordered by bare branches. The prince's golden pate catches the sun and seems to have been set on fire, a warming beacon on a winter's day. The statue was restored in the 1990s and renewed in gold leaf after eighty long years of being daubed in black paint.

Looking around me, there seems to be a certain formality to Kensington Gardens, an almost business-like way of walking dogs and pushing prams. I try to climb down but am wracked with pins and needles; if you spend long periods sitting in the tree tops your legs cease to respond to your central nervous system. After much stretching I land back on park soil and visit the tree's inverted brother, a weeping beech intertwining pendulous arms with a neighbouring cedar. The 'upside-down' tree is an odd sight bereft of its leaves, a tangle of thin branches like a discarded wig.

The High Bower, Greenwich Park
Cedrus atlantica/Atlas cedar

In Greenwich Park, lines of oaks march up the hill from the riverside academy like naval cadets, unerring in their course. I stray across undulating lawns, away from the crowds flocking around the observatory, and up the park's western boundary with Crooms Hill Road through a field of yellowed long grass. High on the bank above me spread the fronds of an Atlas cedar.

I'm panting as I come up under the tree, which leans back sedately against the incline of the hill. The cedar derives its name from its native mountains in Morocco and Algeria, and the parched grass of August provides a suitable backdrop. Bereft of a friend to lift me into the join of the lower reaches, I'm forced to climb a branch like a rope strung between dockside and ship, hand over hand, ankles locked over the top. Once up in the tree I circumnavigate the first ring of limbs, bridging the gaps and feeling like a cartoon character stretched over impossible drops.

Reaching the south side, I follow a diversion up an outstretched arm to a small fork. At the axis an old wound is revealed, the dial of an amputated limb puckered at the edges where the bark has healed. I try counting the rings on its face but give up, losing track at forty.

Squirrels quarrel in the crown of a neighbouring sweet chestnut and one jumps the void between the two trees, springing from the end of a branch and landing a few feet over my head. A second follows in hot pursuit but pulls up short at the sight of me. The runaway, with great agility, has already vanished into the cedar's far side, having seized the opportunity to make good its escape. The second squirrel can only sit clicking its tongue at me with impotent rage, and after a minute or two of this stalemate it turns tail and performs the same remarkable manoeuvre in reverse, flying into the neighbouring crown.

I crawl back to the trunk. The bark has warmed in the heat of the day, and cedar needles have turned pale yellow in death, fallen into cracks between its scales. Reaching the next tier, I pause, high up against the east side of the tree. A small crossing branch between me and the drop acts like the safety bar on a fairground pirate ship, and the view falls away downhill. The golden weathervane of the naval college flashes in the sun and planes headed for City Airport shave dockland skyscrapers as they descend.

On the summit of the hill behind the cedar is Henry Moore's sculpture *Standing Figure: Knife Edge*. It has wandered the length of the nation since it was first installed here in 1979, spending several years in Moore's native Yorkshire before returning to its plinth. Today it seems as if it hasn't budged for a thousand years, much like the gnarled ancients of Greenwich Park, sweet chestnuts whose bellies have swollen with age. I make my exit through the Flower Garden, another conifer paradise in which a child high in a pine tree throws cones at his hapless friends.

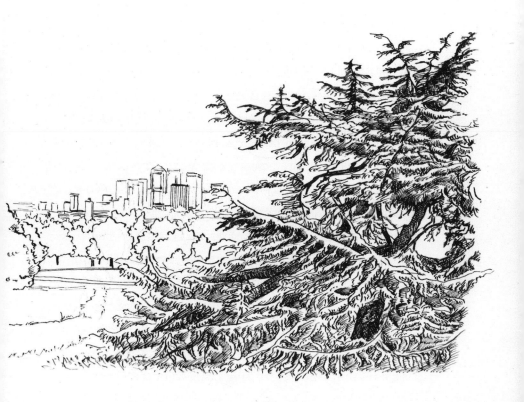

The Royal Perch, St James's Park
Taxodium distichum/Swamp cypress

If, like the author, your chances of taking tea with the Queen are slim, you can indulge in the next best thing, an audience with Buckingham Palace from the summit of neighbouring St James's Park.

At the park's west end, facing the wedding cake of the royal residence, stand two giant trees. Imports from America's Deep South, these twin swamp cypresses have been drinking London lake water for ninety years.

Of the two, the tree to the south of the lake provides the easier ascent. Making my way across the Blue Bridge, I nimbly dodge trains of tourists force-feeding ducks. Once on the south side I follow the water west towards the palace.

The swamp cypress is hard to miss, standing head and shoulders above its neighbouring trees, straight-backed as a palace guard. The climber is rarely conspicuous, but to avoid an audience I carefully time my approach. The lowest branch is within easy reach; once I've gained this and climbed a little higher, I am hidden from the crowds and pause to admire the strange pink hue of the tree in which I sit.

The bark on the trunk has a stringy texture, smoothing in places to a paper consistency. Looking up, I see a rosy stairway spiralling above me for seventy feet, the branches closely spaced with plentiful holds. The thicker arms grow in a helix; ascending, I follow these around the trunk as if climbing a church tower. Before long I'm well above the ice-cream

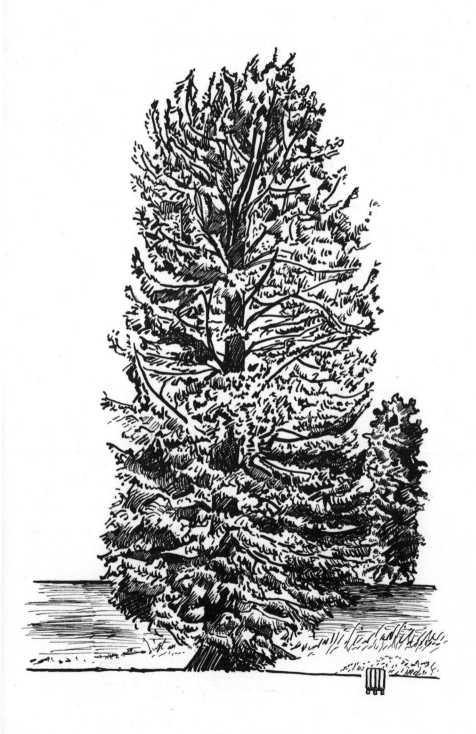

crowds, peep holes in the summer foliage revealing a network of paths below.

At the tree's peak, four branches fan out like the twisted prongs of a fork. Sitting at their junction, I have a comfortable saddle for my legs and a strong support for my back. To the south the tiny capsules of the London Eye can be seen revolving in silence. In front and far below the toy soldiers of Buckingham Palace parade between pill boxes and Russian pelicans glide along the length of the lake. The sound of taxis and cyclists waging war on The Mall filters through a canopy of green needles, soon to turn cinnamon orange with autumn. Unlike most other conifers, this giant will drop its leaves at the end of the year, living up to its nickname, the 'bald cypress'.

I descend the spiral in reverse, returning to planet earth like a newborn god. Exiting the tree's shadow, I try not to startle the man asleep on the adjacent bench.

The Tree of Knowledge, Richmond Park
Fagus sylvatica/Common beech

This vast arena on the fringe of central London is neither open country nor city park. Walking in the shade of ancient oaks, I emerge abruptly on to a network of tarmac roads that divides the park like a sundial. Herds of red deer twitch in the long grass and jumbo jets hoover the sky overhead.

In a park with twelve hundred ancient trees – never mind the rest – the climber is in danger of overdose. I wind my way south across three and a half square miles of parkland, stopping to scale a solitary oak. I spend more time prostrate than aloft, worshipping at the feet of unclimbable giants, in awe of their size and age. The names of Richmond's groves etch themselves on the memory: Kidney Wood, Killcat Corner, Two Storm Wood, Bone Copse, Kings Clump.

At the southern end of Isabella's Plantation, lost and trying to find a way out, I discover the beech by chance. Its bizarre

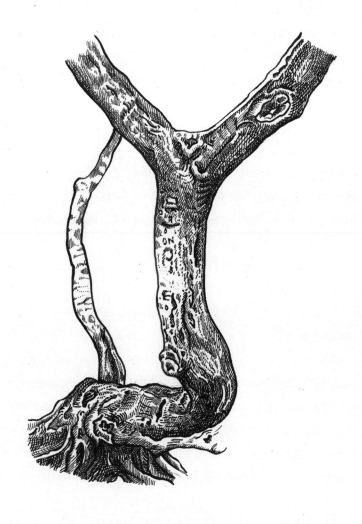

growth stops me in my tracks; never did a tree look more serpentine than this, with five arms rising from a low bole like a coiling mass of snakes. The formation is so unusual it can only be the result of human intervention – the heavy coppicing of years gone by. Everywhere the thin skin of the beech is etched with dark scars, crossed hearts old and new.

The southern arm rears up with all the menace of a hooded cobra, splitting at its peak into two symmetrical branches, the fork of a hissing tongue. Climbing onto the north–south axis of the snake's belly, I walk towards this rearing head. The smooth bark defies grip but, stretching up, I find a ring of wood hidden in the fork. I heave myself up the serpent's neck and out over its open jaws.

Hanging from the join, I feel little sense of being supported by anything at all. Looking back down the length of the beech at its wicked tail end, I think of the first serpent to uncoil from the forbidden tree and tempt Eve into sin. A latter-day Adam and Eve stroll past arm and arm, arguing loudly about which way to go.

The Lookout, Primrose Hill
Quercus robur/English oak

Where the hill begins to rise on the north-west side of the park I make a beeline for a spreading oak. The trunk is bleeding rainwater from a hole in its midriff and the bottom branch has been polished to a dull yellow by past climbers. Well-worn oak takes on an almost plastic quality, like imitation wood in a theme park. Near the roots what looks like 'Otis' has been scrawled on the bark, and I try picturing the Georgia native writing his follow-up to '(Sittin' on) The Dock of the Bay' reclining in the branches.

A false summit twenty feet up the tree has the best outlook, a shaggy, leaf-lined window giving on to central London. Through this circular opening I can see neat pathways dividing the park and the netted enclosure of London Zoo's aviary framing the airspace behind. Flashes of tropical colour contrast with the leaden city skyline, and I think of other enclosures in the zoo, like the plastic mountain of the Mappin Terraces, where bears roam high above the city.

Continuing up the oak, I'm forced to make a daring last move on smaller branches to gain the highest seat. I lean back beneath a thick canopy of leaves, the food for a hundred different species of moth.

Looping back down to the ground, I find assorted rubbish littering the roots: the empty sheaths of a Calippo and a used condom.

On the far side of the hill a grove of oaks appears to be regenerating naturally, waist-high saplings unmolested in the shade of their forebears. Climbing one of the parent trees, I draw level with the bald crown of Primrose Hill, where a group of Italian schoolchildren are taking photographs of the view. Looking back towards north London, I see a white tower rising through the leaves; beneath me sunlight filters through branches covered in watery-grey lichen, and I find it hard to bring the ground back into focus through the haze.

Houdini's Door, Regent's Park

Pinus radiata/Monterey pine

I cross into Regent's Park from the west side, skirting the boating lake. Couples ply the water with joyful, mistimed strokes, and ducks glide serenely along the water's edge. On a dark winter's afternoon just shy of a hundred and fifty years ago, a very different scene would have greeted the

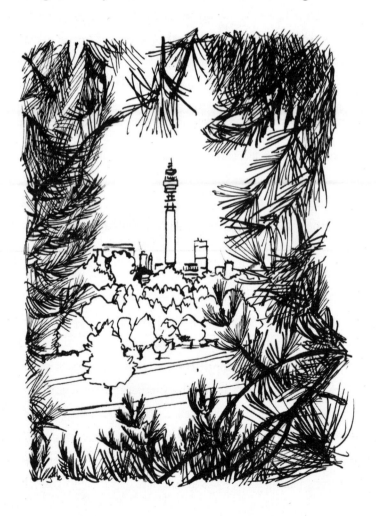

passer-by. On 15 January 1867 two hundred skaters fell into the lake when the ice cracked under them. Weighed down by their blades and cumbersome clothing, forty of them died in the freezing water.

With this morbid thought lingering in the sunshine, I make my way to the far side of the park and then down the Broad Walk to where it meets Chester Road. A group of narcoleptic men smoke and play cards beneath a stand of pines, dozing in turn to allow the game to grind on. I choose the most easterly of the trees, and with an easy step-up on low branches I am soon invisible.

A twisting, corkscrew ascent leads me up through bunched cones that ring the branches like bracelets. To the north I catch a glimmer of gold from the park gates and the paved road of the Inner Circle.

The tree seems to be growing webbed fingers, bark having congealed between splayed branches, creating platforms for the climber. Just below the crown a gap opens in the foliage to reveal a framed view of the BT Tower, the massive hospital blocks of Warren Street marching away behind it. In the foreground the park's pathways lie empty, save for a lone man dragging a suitcase on wheels.

Above a final crosshatch of branches the needles are wet as I push my head through the canopy. Instead of emerging to a panorama I find myself cocooned, a bowl of pine ringing me on all sides. A strong, resin-scented breeze rifles through them and I feel completely hidden, wrapped around in an oversized cloak. This is a tree in which to vanish, and the city has ceased to exist in any tangible way. At ease in this private vault, the climber can happily imagine themselves in the forest vastness of Siberia or the Rocky Mountains.

Across the park someone is practising a trumpet. The notes are so clear I feel like the player is sitting in a nearby tree top, level with my own perch. There's no tune, but I lie back on the branch bed and let the brass echo drown out jets passing overhead. From the tree's base my legs must look cut off, a torso already halfway to heaven, and I linger before dropping back through the canopy and down to the world of men.

Streets, Roundabouts & Rooftops

Trees can be found alive and well in places where other plant life has long since succumbed. In parts of the city they have become the last strongholds of the natural world, lone warriors on roadsides or under flyovers, long forgotten in the midst of roundabouts and refuse sites, everything else having been fenced in or out.

This chapter is a tribute to these solitary trees, clinging to the soil under the city's streets and surviving in its odd corners. It is a daily struggle fraught with peril. Growing on the front line, their bark – painted black by a cocktail of pollution – is livid with scars, their branches clipped by high-sided lorries and their roots salted by winter spreaders.

Without the security of fenced acres their fate is in the hands of councils and developers. Few street trees are safeguarded by preservation orders where space is at a premium; if you search London's planning portals you will find long lists of the doomed, permissions sought and granted to fell.

Trees also contend with human waste. In the city our street surfaces are colonised by litter, and each piece attracts the next. Give people two railings with a narrow enough gap between, and a line of bottles, cigarette packets and plastic cartons will quickly accrue. Wherever litter can be shoved, squeezed or wedged it will gather in every available crevice. Young saplings fall prey to this phenomenon, drowning in a sea of rubbish that rises inside their own guard rails. In the same way, trees with deep boles present attractive receptacles; it is amazing what you can discover festering within. I've climbed into horse chestnuts knee deep in aluminium cans, and found oaks with the bones of fried chicken locked between branch and trunk.

Bark absorbs heavier discards over time. If you opened the trunks of old roadside trees the most extraordinary objects might be found within. There is an oak in a Suffolk hamlet that has swallowed an entire bicycle, its owner having abandoned it against the trunk a hundred or more years ago. The spokes and handlebars still project from the bole and the rusted bell remains attached, although it no longer chimes. No doubt some of London's old trees have more macabre contents, blunt knives and bones buried deep in heartwood.

* * *

The legacy of those that have lost their battle is traced in our maps. Pick up an A–Z of the city, leaf through its index and you will find countless roads, avenues and thoroughfares bearing the names of our native trees. Many are the oak and ash streets I've journeyed down in the hope of finding familiar branches, only to encounter waste bins, drainage holes and unbroken kerbs. Where are the silver stems on Beech Street, now a road tunnel beneath the Barbican's towers? Along Pine Street in neighbouring Clerkenwell the 'Scotch Fir' was felled long ago, and there's no shade for the weary commuter. No limes grow on Lime Street and no russet fruit hangs from the cold façades of Apple Tree Yard. Saddest of all are Elm Grove, Elm Road and Elm Way, diseased streets unlikely to ever reseed their own history. Long gone are the nine elms of Vauxhall; so too the Seven Sisters, the famous siblings that once grew so tall in Tottenham.

In a city as old and dense as London, none of this is very surprising. New planting schemes will seed other byways and trees will flourish elsewhere, even as our choices are dictated by a new underground bureaucracy; electrical wires, gas lines and fibre-optic cables given priority over living roots. Where the street tree struggles on it gives welcome relief to eyes tired of stone and steel. The roadside canopy provides a vital green accent in a grey kingdom, a reminder of another world that existed before the one we inhabit.

Rare trees have even benefited from urban isolation. The famous Marylebone Elm is the last of its genus to survive in central London, saved from the scourge of Dutch elm disease, which killed twenty-five million trees in Britain. Bounded by concrete and with no close neighbours, this elm was spared from bark beetles carrying the deadly fungus and cross-contamination from roots intertwined underground.

Good climbing on the city's roadsides is hard to find. Councils 'limb up' trees so that they don't touch cars or interfere with thoroughfares. When chanced upon, however, street trees offer the climber the purest escape of all. Rising above gum-spotted pavements and clogged intersections, we journey up and over the rubbish of our modern living.

This chapter is also a search for trees sprouting in the dead spaces of the city: the mysterious circles of urban roundabouts, cordoned no man's land where human feet rarely tread, years passing with only wind-blown objects crossing from one side to the other; incongruous rooftop trees, embedded in the thin lips of tower blocks and living on an altogether different plane.

In spite of all the perils with which these isolated trees contend, they continue to burrow beneath and blossom above us, even as we raise the city higher around them. Pay your respects to these brave outposts of bark and branch, persisting on ground long ceded to the city.

The One-Way Willow,
Swiss Cottage Roundabout

Salix × sepulcralis/White weeping willow

Heading north on Loudoun Road, I see a roundabout with
a willow spread across its middle. A quick sprint between
passing lorries and the way to the tree is signed; a set of
stone steps breaks the wall encircling the roundabout and
invites me up, as if to a long-standing monument.

The willow is bedraggled, a wet mop of a tree hiding its
face from the traffic. I duck in under the sweep of leaves and

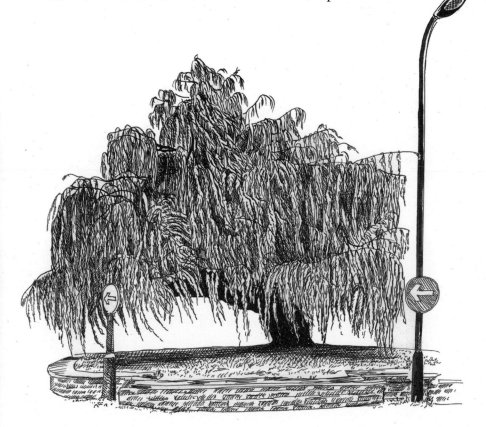

run up the sloping side of the trunk. Slouching against a thick branch, I watch as a van and a red scooter narrowly avoid colliding on the road. A hasty exchange of middle fingers follows before they part ways again. Seen from the heart of the willow, the constant intersecting of traffic is like a badly choreographed dance.

An irksome itch at my elbow leads to the discovery of a large ant colony. On further inspection the tree has been occupied from root to crown, thousands of ants climbing in curving procession. Following their trail, I move around the back of the trunk, trying to grab the next branch while hanging from the arse end of the willow. Over-eager at the thought of a bird's-eye view, I slip, falling to the ground in the middle of the roundabout. Pride and coccyx are bruised, but my embarrassment turns to wonder on spotting a gem of a beetle on my forearm. Subsequent research identifies it as a 'rose chafer'; its metallic-green sheen would dull the emeralds of any London jeweller.

Two teenagers swing by beneath the tree, arm in arm. The boy gestures, saying, 'We used to climb this,' but his companion is uninterested and neither of them look up. Leaving the willow, I enter a shop on the west side of the roundabout advertising Iranian 'khaviar' and buy a paper. The front page describes a man living in a tree on an island in the Thames, accompanied by a photograph of a very respectable-looking pensioner cocooned in a hammock.

Tramp's Corner, The Mall
Platanus × acerifolia/London plane

The rain is hammering central London into submission and the only souls brave enough to remain on the streets have military-grade umbrellas, the kind that repel lightning strikes.

I walk east down The Mall, the brooding hulk of Buckingham Palace crouched at my back. Mature London planes parade alongside me, sweeping the squall into my eyes. None of these proud Victorians is climbable, their lowest branches sprouting at the height of a cavalryman's plumed helmet.

Just before reaching the shelter of Admiralty Arch, I pass a cloister of younger trees, three planes rooted on the north side of the road, their branches spilling onto the doorstep of the Ugandan Embassy. They seem to huddle together in the downpour, as do a group of homeless men on the stone bench behind them, their sleeping bags like sponges in the flood.

The nearest plane has sharp elbows close to the ground. Pollarding has given its branches a clumsy aspect, like a tree tripping over itself. I jump and lock my hands in the joint, swinging a sodden leg over the branch. Patches of flaked bark have turned bright yellow in the rain, while the older layer has blackened; the effect is of a spotted python unravelling from above.

I sit on the west-facing arm, my back against the tree and the rainwater running out of my trouser leg like a spout. The world beyond the crown is lost in a veil of rain ricocheting off the road. I can hear some plucky birds tuning up across The Mall in St James's Park, not that anyone is lingering to listen.

Sliding back down to the ground, I am surrounded by Empire. Nelson soars above Trafalgar Square, and next to the three planes is a memorial to Royal Marines slain far from home in the wilds of rural China.

Less imperial is one of the surviving 'Seven Noses of Soho' under the arch, a 1990s installation by an artist peeved at the city-wide introduction of CCTV. Dodge a taxi or two, and you can jump up and stroke it for good luck.

The Spire, Highbury Island
Pinus radiata/Monterey pine

I arrive at Highbury Island just before dawn on a Sunday morning. Traffic across the three lanes of the roundabout is light and a squirrel squats obstinately in the middle of the road. I watch a police car turn lazily up Canonbury Road before I cross the tarmac and leap the fence.

Under the cover of conifers the patchy lawn has an abandoned air and there's no sign of other trespassers. I look east towards a weak sunrise beginning to filter through the canopy. Standing on this same spot seventy-one years ago, I would have seen a shadow cross the sun, the deadly silhouette of a V-1 flying bomb. On 27 June 1944 Highbury Corner suffered a direct hit, killing twenty-six people and injuring

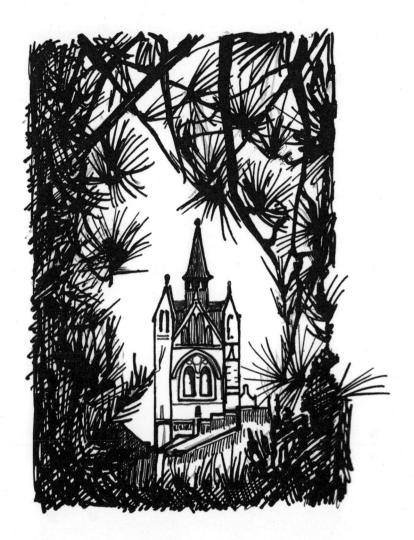

another hundred and fifty. The roundabout was laid out in the 1960s on the site of this former devastation, although most of the trees look considerably younger, and the circle mimics the old extent of Compton Terrace Gardens, now confined to the east side of Upper Street.

Dominating the island is a Monterey pine. I step up into the lowest branches and the air feels three degrees warmer, thick with a strong scent of resin, a respite from the reek of Islington's Saturday-night leftovers.

Ascending, I place my hands on separate branches, a chest breadth apart, before elevating myself to the next tier like a vertical oarsman. Near the summit the trunk twists and bends outward, and the last few branches are a nervous step-ladder poised over the drop. I hoist myself through the pine's thick head of hair and emerge, high above the other round-about trees, at the pinnacle of my own small forest. The twig ends of the crown are ringed in tiny pine cones, understudies of the cone-bearing branches below.

To the south the Gothic Revival tower of Union Chapel is set in a thick frame of pine needles. Damaged by the doodle-bug and struck twice by lightning, its brick and mortar has weathered a difficult century. Directly ahead of me the Holloway Road is a grey tract far below, surfed by model white vans through miniature roadworks.

An hour later I emerge from the shadow of the round-about and climb back over the fence, leaving the island behind, a rare sanctuary in the turmoil of central London.

The Burnt Treehouse, Lillie Road
Platanus × acerifolia/London plane

On the edge of the West Kensington Estate a strip of green borders the roadside. A London plane stands alone on this solitary patch, looking abject at its isolation. A deep hollow has been carved out at the bottom of the trunk below ground level, the kind of place you might stash stolen goods or state secrets.

A scrap of jaundiced paper hangs by a single nail to the bark. Stained by months – or possibly years – of weather, it is hard to decipher. After much scrutiny it appears to be an advertisement for a local clairvoyant called Richard. The stand-out quote reads, 'The artwork was channelled from the highest source to provide healing mandala focus for better health and wealth. Shogun treasure!' The paper is slit at the bottom with a row of phone numbers. None have been torn off.

A long, bare midsection forces me to wedge my hands, one on top of the other, on a single branch and make a jump for the next. The remains of wooden planks, once nailed to the tree to serve as steps, have rotted away and provide no purchase.

Up in the crown I am surrounded by the charred ruins of an old treehouse. Golden sweet wrappers, Werther's Originals, are all that remain of whatever summits were once held here. Perhaps Richard used to sit in this makeshift den, palm reading in the sky.

The Flying Oak, Kensington Roof Gardens
Quercus robur/English oak

The lift's golden doors give onto an empty restaurant, a lone waiter polishing glass at the counter. Behind him a corridor slopes down to an open doorway and a glimpse of green borders beyond.

I've come to the Roof Gardens on a rare morning when they lie open to the public. First laid out in the 1930s as an escape from the city, today the gardens are more often in use for private events. Under a sullen sky I have the whole acre and a half to myself.

In the 'English Woodland Garden' a shallow watercourse is bounded by a brick wall, preventing it from cascading onto Derry Street six floors below. Portholes in the brick coursing, like the eyepieces of telescopes, reveal far-reaching views over London, and the grey Goliath of the Kensington Holiday Inn is perfectly framed through ornamental ironwork.

Flamingos stand knee-deep in the model river, blinking at me without interest. Their wings are not clipped, and I picture pink UFOs taking off from the parapet and sailing out across High Street Kensington. Apparently the birds are free to escape but choose not to; the eldest has been resident here for over sixteen years. They have become institutionalised, content to rule their rooftop domain.

Three ivy-wrapped oaks are spaced at even intervals across the south-facing lawn. The trees date from the original gardens and are over seventy years old – they were already saplings during the Blitz. Growing in just eighteen inches of soil, their shallow root balls spread laterally and have been carefully cultivated by the garden's overseers. I wonder how the atmospheric condition of the Roof Gardens compares with the city's parks far below.

The most westerly of the three oaks is a modest height for its age, although it does begin a hundred feet above the street. I leave my shoes in a flowerbed, with the flamingos eyeing them longingly, and climb onto the first branch with due care (all three oaks are listed under tree preservation orders). The limbs are widely spaced and my feet slip in their ivy cloak, but before long I emerge head first from the canopy.

Standing with my feet in the tree's upper fork, I hang above London. I have become a character in one of my favourite childhood books, *The Tale of the Land of Green Ginger*, in which a mythical floating garden flies across the deserts of Arabia, settling at random every night in a new location. Surveying the city from the oak's canopy, I stand in a real-world incarnation of a magical oasis.

The Soldier Fig, Stratford Greenway
Ficus carica/Common fig

In 2010 *Time Out* published *The Great Trees of London*. This noble tome recorded some of the city's most loved trees: the fattest, tallest, oldest and strangest. In among famed giants and ancient boles was a curious anomaly – a common fig growing by the side of a dual carriageway. In spite of being listed as a 'great tree', no plaque was affixed to the spot and no future assured. The author, Jenny Landreth, concluded that the tree would be lucky to survive the building sites piling up on every side.

Five years late I decide to go in search of this fabled fig tree and find out if it still clings to its precarious hold on the city; an ulterior motive is that I'm very fond of eating figs. Cycling down the four-lane High Street, I pull off at a gate to the Greenway, a path running through Newham and Stratford towards the Olympic Park.

A giant new housing development looms overhead and the footpath is barred with steel mesh. Peering through the lattice, I can just make out a clutch of fig leaves poking above the parapet of a footbridge. I retrace my steps and cross the Waterworks River on a bridge leading to Otter Close. The footpath is barred here, too, but I sneak into the private car park and hop over some low railings. Ahead a short, over-grown track leads back up the waterside to the fig, now visible as a great cascade tumbling onto the footpath.

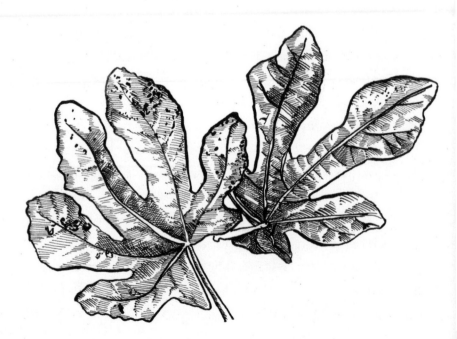

The fig is a tree to climb into, not up. I wrestle my way through a bramble bush and into the tree's silver-stemmed understorey. Multiple shoots spring up from between car tyres and old bricks, surrounded by a host of dog collars, Frisbees and beer cans. A glut of unharvested fruit hangs overhead and I pull a dozen figs down off the tree. A vigorous rub cleans off their outer layers of grime and I bite into the pick of the bunch – not quite ripe but still delicious. All around the air is filled with the sounds of jack-knifing, slab splitting and wire cutting, but I lie hidden in the heart of the tree with no other company than a few fruit-drunk wasps.

Such an incongruous hideaway was well worth the journey, the bramble cuts and the demonic stare I receive from a man in a hard hat on my way back down the canal. Like Landreth before me, I wonder if this fig will still be fighting its corner in years to come.

Pedalling home, I stop at a Sainsbury's in Stratford. I cruise the fruit aisle and find a small, slightly squashed pack of Turkish figs priced at £2. They bear poor comparison to the local crop I ferry home in my pocket.

Seasons

Generations pass while some tree stands, and old
families last not three oaks.

Urne-Burial, Sir Thomas Browne

Climb a mountain twice and the landscape remains
unchanged. Snows come and go, but the bedrock is steadfast
and the peaks retain their timeless cast. Climb a tree and
return a few months later, and the transformation is marked;
growth, decline and the cycle of the seasons make no two
ascents the same.

Trees frame our cities and the changes they undergo
throughout the year affect our impression of the whole.

What markers of the seasons would we have bereft of them, glass and concrete marking neither the passage of winter nor the coming of spring? Trees anchor us in nature's cycle; lining our pavements and filling our parks, they remind us of another kind of time-keeping, a vegetable clock that keeps ticking to an alternative rhythm.

In spring the existence of the city's plant life makes itself tangibly felt among us again. Sap begins to flow in the veins of deciduous trees, and the climber feels the draw of new growth and a desire to revisit old roosts. The sudden surge of vegetation is a wake-up call after the long months of winter, and the arrival of leaves on gaunt branches transforms the urban landscape, impacting our sight lines and reconfiguring our streets. One moment we're looking through the bars of a gate, the next it has turned into a solid green wall, the city's hard edges softened by budding crowns.

Returning to a favourite perch, we feel it stretch out winter cramps with buds breaching the bark and everything pushing outward. Before long the flowers of horse chestnuts, maples, oaks and others emerge. Squirrels surface from tree-top drays and birds build new nests or return to the old. The world above and below the tree comes to life, a cornucopia of wildlife awaiting its rebirth. The transformation of trees in spring is a green injection to the city's stone-grey heart.

In summer, heat alters our perception once more; the trees rise like balloons, while the hot corridors of the city sweat down below. There is no better place than the canopy when high summer settles on the city – ground-dwelling folk itch inside buttoned-up shirts, sweat beading on foreheads and running down necks, while stale air stagnates in offices and Undergrounds. Up in the branches the breeze seems to come from far afield, carrying a trace of Arcadian air and lifting the mantle of the tree. It is a sonorous wind, bringing boughs and leaves to life, and shaking whole streets out of their stupor. Without the trees the city would not twitch at all, the blank face of the man-made sitting dumb and inert.

A tree in full leaf is the perfect hideaway. Stepping into the shade of an oak or beech, the climber reaches up to grab hold of a branch and disappears into a ceiling of green. The canopy provides solitude from the street, and sitting in this thin band of green we are of neither earth nor sky, suspended between two elements. Residing in the cool shade of a hundred thousand leaves, climbers are rewarded with their own floating summerhouse.

As a child I remember jumping from a ledge into a waterfall in Sutherland and being pushed down, driven by the cascade into the deep sinkhole under the falls. At first all was chaos and white water; I couldn't swim to the surface and began struggling in panic. Then I opened my eyes and found myself in a silent emerald room, a still bowl carved out of the rock by millions of years of falling water. It was a moment of absolute clarity that lasted a heartbeat, before the river's current picked me up and brought me back to the surface. I am reminded of this experience perched in summer trees, each cavernous interior a green room of its own.

At the tail end of summer a city's foliage becomes flat and exhausted. All the lustre of spring has long gone and the leaves are wilted, turned in on themselves. The city's dust has settled on jaded canopies and every tree appears mummified. This embalming brings with it an expectancy of change, and before long a second wave of colour sweeps the city.

As deciduous trees suspend their food production and prepare for winter, chlorophyll is withdrawn from the leaves and other pigments are revealed. Every species has its own spectrum and every leaf turns by degrees. Copper and bronze, coral and crimson, fawn, hazel, gold and umber, autumn leaves outshine spring flowers. Ascending through these tunnels of colour, the climber is draped in a finer coat than any adorning shoulders far below.

From the vantage point of a tree's crown we can watch the way different leaves fall to the ground, end over end, spiralling sideways or descending in tight, sculpted circles. The five-lobed leaf of the London plane drops away like a rocking horse, swaying back and forth on the draught, while beech leaves plummet to earth, flailing as they fall. Other leaves cartwheel or descend with the graceful arcs of a paper aeroplane carried far from the roots of the tree. Each charts its own course into the wind.

Trees remove their shrouds at differing speeds. Some seem to drop one leaf at a time, while others fall like water dripping from a tap. Then there are those that cast off their burden in a single shrug. The ginkgo retains all its leaves at sundown but is bare in the dawn light, an overnight dump spread around the roots like a bed of yellow gold. On still days, when falling leaves seem to be the only moving parts of the scenery, we climb as if locked in slow motion with a world in transition around us. Reaching the apex of a branch, we can pluck the final leaf, still clinging to the twig.

The fruits of trees also begin to detach. The climber is surrounded by seeds dispersing on different flight paths; the twin wings of sycamores split and spinning, or strands of falling ash keys. Autumn ascents through horse chestnut and oak are accompanied by the soft soundtrack of nuts falling into the leaf litter; conkers unlocked and acorns plummeting to the floor, soon to be seized by squirrels.

When the last leaves have fallen but are not yet collected or scattered by street cleaners and gardeners' rakes, their patterns make a kaleidoscope when viewed from above. Thousands of tonnes are shed across the city, accumulating in drifts like the disassembled pieces of an enormous jigsaw. This colourful array drains the landscape all around and focuses the climber's eye on the intricate carpet beneath them. Autumn is the most reflective time to be in the trees; the smoky season briefly slows the pace of the city, and the sense of seasonal change is never more acute.

The short days and hard frosts of winter might not seem the ideal time to go and perch in a tree and, for many, autumn is the climber's swan song. The warm cocoon of summer leaves is long gone on all but the evergreens, and the trees reveal their bare bones. Walking through a park on a December day, it can be hard to recognise familiar faces, the fat green giants of July reduced to skeletal form. If you have ever owned and washed a cat you will know a similar shock – a great fluff ball reduced to a wraith in the flash of a shower head. Climbing trees in the dark months of winter is not for the timid or shy. There's no reassuring layer of leaves between us and the iron-hard ground. Hanging on high branches, we stand exposed to the elements and people passing beneath.

Yet winter's nakedness brings with it a cleansing aura and a new clarity of light. What we lose in cover, we gain in views; the city is revealed in its totality through branches wrapped in hoarfrost. Though hands might freeze to bark and cold weather make for slippery climbs, winter's aerial perspective is worth the effort needed to attain it.

The season's exposed latticework also reveals the individual majesty of branches. Where summer drapery hides the summit, winter allows the climber to plot a far-reaching route from the ground. To climb a tree in your mind, before ever setting foot in its branches, is a powerful exercise in imagination, following the tracery of crowns and judging the scale and slope of each branch. Can a gap be bridged and a perch reached? Like a mountaineer pointing at ice fields far above, so we can stand beneath the black outline of a winter tree and envisage the climb to come.

John Donne wrote of a December day, 'The world's whole sap is sunk.' When looking down on a frozen park from above, this sense of nature withdrawing from the city is everywhere evident. The trees stand stark and immutable even as the machinery of the street keeps turning.

The rare day when a blizzard blows through the city is an enchanted time to be in the trees, the black and white contrast of snow and bark reducing the world to a chequerboard. While snow on the street quickly turns to sludge –

scraped with shovels and sprayed with salt – in the clasp of branches it settles like white moss. Park, garden and riverside are almost deserted, and the snow dampens the sounds of traffic. If you venture into a fir or pine, the snowfall lies heavy on thick needles, a shaggy coat for the climber.

If we travel through the year in the company of trees, we gain an intimate knowledge of their anomalies. Close to my front door in Whitechapel is a London plane whose branches cross hands with the steel arm of a street light. Climbing through its crown in December, I find all its leaves have fallen bar one small crop, growing hard against the light's plastic mantle. As the days shorten, trees across the city shed their burden to conserve energy; with insufficient sunlight for photosynthesis, leaves drop off and the trees enter a period of dormancy. But the street light's halogen bulb has tricked the plane into retaining this fistful of leaves, the false sun confusing its natural timekeeping. A few weeks later this may lead to frost damage, the remaining leaves preventing the bark from sealing itself against the advent of winter weather. The seasonal cycle of the tree has been altered by the microclimate of an urban space.

Living in the city we easily become separated from the natural world. The trees provide a vital lifeline, and their adherence to an older pattern of living can reconnect us all. While spring returns to some cities, autumn comes to others, and our counterpart climbers on the far side of the world navigate bare branches as we wade through fresh growth. In the city we should cleave to what vestiges we have of natural time, not the abstraction of office hours or the sensors of street lights. In the words of the Welsh poet R. S. Thomas:

> *Space and time*
> *Are not the mathematics that your will*
> *Imposes, but a green calendar*
> *Your heart observes.*

Where better to remember this than in the evolving arms of a tree?

Open Ground

We approach a wilder sensibility when exploring spaces that lack concerted cultivation. In the suburbs of many towns and cities a rift appears where buildings break like the tide on vast fields of upland and lowland, marshland and scrub. These are the bald patches in the urban mane, swathes of land criss-crossed for centuries. They follow no single plan or rule of design, and the essential character of each is different.

If you set out to explore these hollow realms, catch an early train and return after dark. You will need all the hours in the day to map their many paths. Some have an abundance of climbing trees, while others only a few lonely towers.

*   *   *

Venturing from city streets onto open ground we experience a sudden scattering; crowds disperse like rice thrown on a kitchen floor. Stepping over the margin of Clapham Common or Hackney Marsh feels like being shoved hard in the back. We are propelled inward, lonely figures moving towards private goals.

This scattering has a deep psychological effect on the visitor. Just as the tunnel of the street becomes claustrophobic, so the relief of open ground is also unsettling. We feel like moving targets after the shelter of a built-up environment.

The city's common land is a bewildering zone, a place in which the unwary are led astray. No longer channelled down familiar walkways, we become easily disorientated. Passers-by are swallowed on the fringe, emerging hours later bemused and bereft of purpose.

All open ground is unstable; disturbed acres dug up and fenced over, hiding innumerable buried objects. The city is only fish-skin thick, and we can peel away its oily surface to reveal older territory beneath. Ancient avenues of sweet chestnuts border fields of rubble from the Blitz, and Roman roads hide beneath a few feet of soil. It's hard for anything to truly impress itself on these spaces. They remain forever no man's land.

Cast adrift on the city's commons and heaths, trees can look a little lost. Huddled in clumps like nervous sheep or frozen alone on the skyline, they stand exposed to the hunter's roving eye. Some are long tired of city living, scarecrows full of dead branches. Others grow proud and tall, leaf-bearing lighthouses that rise high above their surroundings. Crossing a half-mile between two climbing trees we get a sense of the untold millions that lie beyond the city limits and the adventures to be had in the great beyond.

The microclimate of the street is dispelled on open ground and clouds convene with the crowns of trees. Instead of looking up at narrow corridors of sky the weather rolls in from every horizon, playing out strange fantasies. When fog comes to the city it settles on these wide acres; sea haars snaking their way up the river to Blackheath and morning mist crowning Hampstead's hilly scalp. These are exposed places, stretches of the city where rain clouds seem to alight and lightning always strikes twice.

Throughout the calendar year common land becomes the staging ground for long-held tradition; the circus that rolls in and out in high summer or the bonfires of November, when Guy Fawkes is immolated across London. There is no better place to watch fireworks in autumn than from a tree, exploding rockets mimicking the canopy in which you sit. All these transitory elements flower then fade, arriving in a riot of colour before leaving the same lonely spaces in their wake.

It is possible to thread our own paths through the trees, inventing maps signposted by a high beech or a twisted oak. Travelling to visit favourite tree tops feels like an act of pilgrimage in these spaces, as if the climber is paying homage to a wooden idol. The fork of a branch deep in the heart of a city common can become a private hideaway. Returning to an old perch, the way up is second nature.

A Strange Vision, Peckham Rye

Pinus radiata/Monterey pine

I come to the common from the east and make straight for a
mighty poplar in open ground. A topless man with the arms
and torso of an action figure is doing pull-ups on rings strung

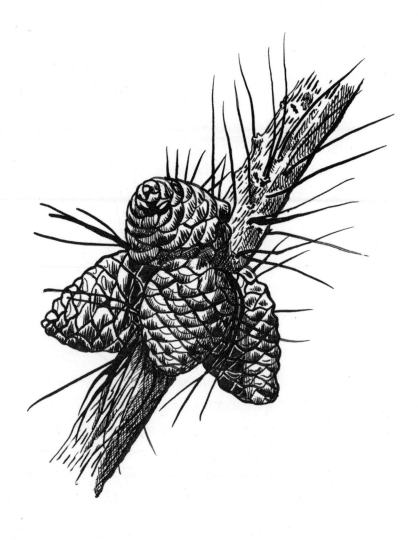

from the lowest branch. We agree that it would be all right for me to climb above him but I give up after ten feet – the poplar precipice is terrifying and violent grunts from below distract from the task at hand.

I wander on, eventually crossing the threshold between common and park, divided by the River Peck, which seems more of a rivulet. Close by the park office is a structure known as 'the Japanese Shelter'; tarred wooden poles project on either side, decorating the ends of this ornamental hut. Behind the shelter is the huge carcass of a felled trunk and beside it a magnificent pine. I sit on the prostrate giant and wait for the walkways to empty before attempting the climb.

As I approach the pine I spy a black fungus that's fallen at its foot. I pick it up, wondering if it's an ill omen. Above me a single branch extends at head height from the south face and I pull myself onto the first rung of the ladder. A squirrel invades from a neighbouring sycamore, then thinks better of it and retreats.

The tree leans ever so slightly to the east. My route takes me from side to side and I find myself climbing an overhang. A woman with a shock of white hair passes thirty feet below and I shy from her upwards glance, hugging the pine's coarse skin.

In the 1760s William Blake crossed Peckham Rye, where he claimed to have had one of his many visions: 'A tree filled with angels, bright angelic wings bespangling every bough like stars'. Perhaps the white-haired woman will report visions of a small, barefoot devil, dropping pine cones like meteorites from above.

The tree is climbable to its full height and the view north over London immense, although partly obscured by the crown of a weeping ash. The long cheese wedge of the common dwindles towards the skyline and the distant towers of the financial district. An area of Peckham Rye briefly served as a prisoner-of-war camp for Italian soldiers during the Second World War. Climbing back down, and eyed suspiciously by a group of speed walkers, I find lunch in an Italian café near to Rye Lane. Maybe its owner's recent forebears once slept out on the common, uncertain what the future might hold.

The Oasis, Blackheath
Populus × canadensis/Hybrid black poplar

The pancake interior of Blackheath offers slim pickings compared with the lush canopy of neighbouring Greenwich Park. Striking out across the heath, I narrowly avoid a two-wheeled blur, a motorbike appearing from nowhere and vanishing in an instant. The echo of its exhaust makes the whole heath seems like a hollow gong for the traffic that dissects it.

Skirting 'Rotten Row', my desperation mounts. I feel like some panicked tree dweller on an empty plain, at a loss for refuge. Even the lamp posts look lonely out here, corridors of them lining the paths as if whole streets have been swept away on either side.

Single trees appear like mirages on the horizon and I make for them, only to find diseased willows or shrub-like alders.

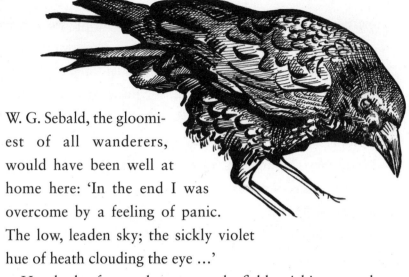

W. G. Sebald, the gloomi-
est of all wanderers,
would have been well at
home here: 'In the end I was
overcome by a feeling of panic.
The low, leaden sky; the sickly violet
hue of heath clouding the eye ...'

Hundreds of crows hop across the fields, picking over the weekend's abandoned picnics and barbecues. One drags the entrails of a pasta dish through tomato-bloodied grass; another two fight over a single eyeball, last of the chicken nuggets. The scene is every bit as grisly as the landscape of a battlefield, carrion stretching in all directions.

I soon get turned around by the paths and lose all sense of orientation. Dark shapes of topless men stalk the peripheries of my vision, gender-neutral breasts shimmering in the heat haze. I stumble in and out of a dried pond and past a ring of gorse bushes, stark amid the acres of grass, perhaps covering one of the fabled mines under Blackheath. I wish that I could find the legendary chalk cavern, turned into a nightclub by rebellious Victorians, with forty steps carved down to its floor and a chandelier hung from the ceiling. A story relates that when it was reopened in 1939 to serve as an air-raid shelter the remnants of the last party ever held there, nearly a century earlier, were found untouched; champagne flutes covered in chalk dust and liquor bottles lining the stone walls.

After what seems like hours of wandering I find a strange sinkhole in the south-west corner of the heath, a verdant escape from its lunar surface. I climb a poplar covered in ivy, its long strands forming a great Rapunzel-like mane. Clinging to its threads, I imagine falling like the knight thrown from the tower and blinded by thorns, but return the way I came without misfortune.

The Turnip Tree, Tooting Commons
Platanus orientalis/Oriental plane

The paths that criss-cross the Commons are shored up by ancient oaks, some of which have been resident for centuries, a last link with the Wildwood that once covered Britain.

Near the northern boundary I find an English oak surrounded by the splintered ends of a sawn-off branch. The mouldy remnants of a rope swing hang down from above and the tree is ringed with red tape.

Walking further in, I am stopped short by a plane tree presiding over a fork in the tracks parallel to Bedford Hill Road. The shape of the trunk is arresting, an enormous wasp's nest rising to a threadbare spray of branches. The bole is bloated like a vast baobab, the water-storing giant of the African savannah, but it is covered in a hoary skin, thickening with the passing years. Up close, the trunk is speckled with projecting nodules like clusters of ginger root.

The only sure path to the crown is a single strand of the tree's comical topknot, stretching to the east and descending to the height of a running jump or a friend's shoulders. I leap for the bridge and resort to the time-honoured monkey-bar technique, hand over hand along its length and back to the trunk. As the gradient rises I swing ankles over the branch for added insurance.

On top of the turnip-like tree is a golden disc, the curious scab of an old wound. Concave, it sits between my legs like a stretched drum, ready to beat a bass note across the open grassland stretching away to the south. It's a comfy seat, a modest twelve feet off the ground, and a good spot from

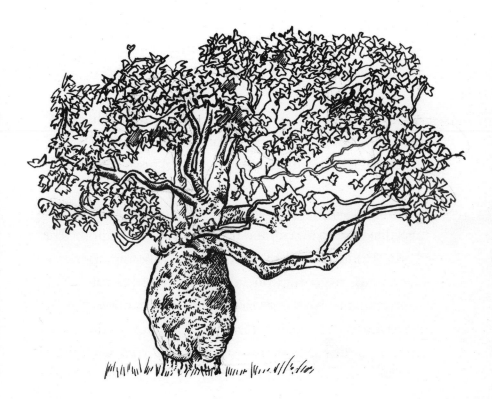

which to watch comings and goings on the Commons. Not so long ago locals would have exercised their shared ownership of the land by putting their animals out here to graze, or digging up the gravel beds under the grass. I watch a mother and child picking blackberries along the roadside, an affirmation of ancient rights.

The pathways beneath the tree are in steady use; joggers, dog walkers and footballers pass under my feet. The plane feels a bit like a toll booth, rooted at an important intersection – perhaps I should demand coin for safe passage. Several people stop and stare up at me, the comical shape of the tree drawing the eye, and I engage in short, stilted conversations. It is an odd sensation being so exposed but inviolate, close to the ground yet far removed. The long bridge into the crown is easily defendable and I spend a happy afternoon guarding my fortress.

Lamp Post 33, Clapham Common
Platanus × *acerifolia*/*London plane*

This is a sad story, a tale of courage found wanting and heights never reached ...

In the middle of Clapham Common's open plains is a ring of gnarled trees, black locusts leaning at odd angles to the ground, their bark wizened and their oval leaves like cutouts from a picture book. They circle London's largest bandstand, a 19th-century cast-iron dome picked out in red and green.

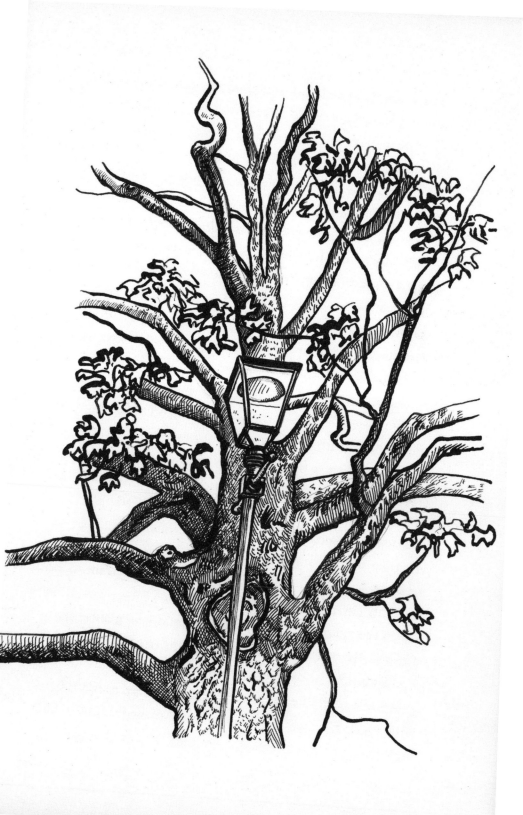

Crossing this magic sphere, I continue down an avenue of London planes marching south towards Balham. The two rows are well established and arch over the path, arms interlacing high above. The trees are interspersed with Victorian lamp posts and the occasional lamp's hood is draped with leaves. They remind me of a lime on Davies Street in Mayfair, which, when in leaf, completely envelops a street light parallel with its trunk. Passing at night, you see a soft emerald glow seeping from under its canopy.

I pause by an intricate crown, a plane with eccentric branches spread in all directions. The lamp post alongside seems to fall just short of the lowest branch, offering a hopeful scaffold to gain the tree. Clasping cold iron in both hands, I place my feet on the beaded ring at the base then haul myself a few feet higher, the whole structure lurching back and forth beneath my weight like a ship's mast in a storm. I reach up and grasp the crossbars, old handholds from an age when lighting gas was a nightly task. The shaking has increased to a Force 8 and the world below is a blur.

I steady myself on the lamp post by crouching and placing my right hand around its coronet top. Leaning out from the lamp like an ungainly Gene Kelly, I find the branch of the tree is further away than I supposed, my fingertips falling just short. The logical next step is to pounce, a short jump from the post to the tree's crown, and I practise flexing my haunches.

A full ten minutes passes in limbo, the lamp post a ridiculous roost for a thirty-year-old man. A mother and child walk hand in hand beneath me, the child loudly asserting that all polar bears are from Poland. Afraid of mockery and filled with regret, I make an ignoble retreat; a leap that would have been second nature to an ape is beyond me, and any confidence evaporates with sickening thoughts of broken bones.

An easier ascent lies in the slice of greensward to the north of Broomwood Road. A squat mushroom of a tree stands with five shattered limbs at its base, evidence of its former glory. The trunk is cut short ten feet off the ground, but all around its waist are the hallmarks of resurrection, a thicket of strong young shoots sprouting like porcupine needles from the bole.

I climb up the south side of this Lazarus tree, a sweet chestnut with a crown of baby hair. Sitting on the sawn-off

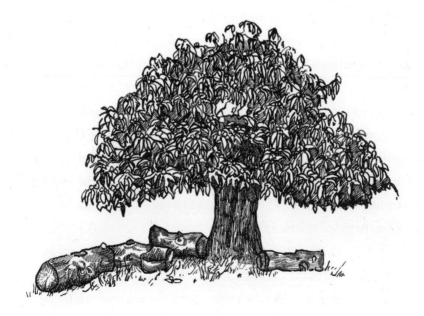

summit, I look down on one of the Common's outdoor gyms. In the warmth of an August evening the pull-up bars and wooden high steps are crowded with muscle men, flexing to the beat of a portable radio.

Gwain's Bane, Wormwood Scrubs
Populus nigra 'Italica'/*Lombardy poplar*

From Scrubs Lane I pass through a thin band of trees and emerge onto a boundless field. The raw scale of the Scrubs is dizzying after the confines of neighbouring streets, and I feel like I have been pushed over the rim of a giant green bowl. In the distance a brooding clump of trees marks the Scrub's woodland copse, a focal point that seems to pull everything irresistibly inward. Rising in its centre are the tall silhouettes of poplars, and I set out with the intent to climb them.

Although walking at a brisk pace, my progress across the Scrubs is negligible; nothing recedes or advances in this vast, empty arena. It was originally designated as a military training ground, but armies assembled here would look like toy soldiers. To the south the skeletal chimney of a hospital incinerator looms over the playing fields, adjoining the eight brick towers of HMP Wormwood Scrubs, a prison built by prisoners from bricks made on site.

Finally I find myself at the tangled feet of the copse. A sense of foreboding hangs over the tunnel-like entrance, where a narrow path has been forced into the middle. The name 'Wormwood' derives from the 15th-century *wormholt-*

wode, 'a snake-infested wood or thicket', and the copse makes a fitting serpent's lair.

The air inside is oppressive. Disturbing totems are trapped in the undergrowth: torn clothing, plastic knives and the body of a decomposed bird. Little light penetrates the ceiling of thorn and the path soon peters out.

I crouch all alone in the centre of a green chapel, half expecting a ghostly axe to come swinging from behind, the Green Knight of Arthurian legend after my head. With no tree to climb and increasingly unsettled, I begin retracing my steps through the tunnel. Without warning a great, snarling sound erupts behind me and I bolt the last ten feet out of the copse. Back in the open air I look up to find my imaginary monster is a toy drone flying overhead.

Circling the wood before leaving, I study a row of fenced spotlights sitting astride portable generators. I wonder if these lights are there to flood the recesses of the copse in the dead of night and flush out evildoers. I leave the park past George Irvin's shut-up funfair – everyone seems to have fled from the Scrubs.

The Talisman, Wandsworth Common
Quercus robur/English oak

The path on the east perimeter of Wandsworth Common is a griddle of exposed tree roots and I watch a cyclist undergo shock therapy as he rides across. I cut west over the Common to the rail lines that bisect it, crossing the bridge by an avenue of London planes. Attached to the brick coursing is a poster advertising 'Ninja Kids', a six-part course certain to turn your child into a killing machine.

My hunt for a good climbing tree leads me to a triangular field south of the lake. Standing alone is an oak with a striking hole in its trunk, like the eye of a cyclops. Closer in, and the hole reveals itself to be a neat, upturned horseshoe of branches, a good augury for the climber.

Clambering up the north face, I gain leverage from a knuckle in the curve of the horseshoe, its bark polished pink with use. A finger-shaped impression in the trunk's bark is the ghost of a lost branch and a trace of viridian paint suggests scrubbed-out graffiti.

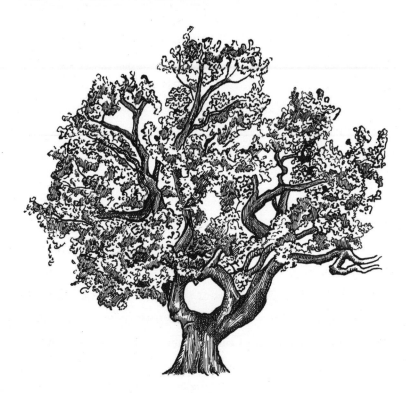

Swinging across one side of the horseshoe, I strike out west to a low perch, but not content with this elevation I start searching for a way onto the upper deck. In the end I am forced to straddle a horizontal branch, legs flailing beneath me as I struggle to pull my body up. The effort is worth the reward and the oak's crown flows on lateral lines, providing endless arms to shuffle out on. There is a curious gap between two parallel limbs, as if the tree is a giant slot machine and by dropping a coin through this cleft every branch will rotate in slow procession.

Errant dogs go speeding by beneath the oak, followed by the imploring shouts of their owners. At one point this common cry becomes a chorus, a bass voice shouting, 'Zippy! Zippy!', while a treble begs 'Umber!' to return. The hopeless servitude of the dogs' owners reminds me of a Kurt Vonnegut short story, in which Thomas Edison's own dog reveals that the entire canine race has willingly subjugated itself to humankind in order to enjoy a life of freeloading. As the spaniel rockets under the tree for the third time, I imagine it laughing to itself, knowing full well its only punishment at day's end will be a bowl of biscuits.

Back on the ground I find curious growths mixed in with the fallen acorns in the leaf litter. Subsequent reading reveals these to be knopper galls, the eggs of small gall wasps that are incubated in the acorns of English oaks, deforming them. Fascinatingly, the gall's two-phase life cycle is only completed by a similar incubation in the male catkins of the Turkey oak – it can only exist where both species of tree are present.

The Commentary Box, Hackney Marshes

Populus tremula/Common 'quaking' aspen

Heading for the marshes up the false arm of the Lee Navigation, I veer from the canal side and into Wick Woodland. A deserted track threads its way between plane trees, and an evil wind, smelling of dead meat, blows through a thicket of tangled ash.

Crossing the Homerton Road, a last line of tree cover gives way to the eighty-eight football fields of Hackney Marshes. Goal posts crowd the middle distance, a hundred and more white gates leading nowhere, and a parrot flash of yellow and green on the horizon marks a huddle of players. Their sporadic calls drift over what the Earl of Meath once called 'the most magnificent playground in the world'.

In the 18th century a great causeway was discovered beneath these fields, cracked stones with Roman coins trodden into the crevices. I traipse the length of another pitch and conjure a legionary alongside me, tramping under the weight of his pack and cursing this godforsaken island.

The marshes are home to a line of native black poplars, an increasingly rare pure breed threatened by the species' habit of forming hybrids with others, and their muddled arms define the margins between playing field and river. Near the East Wood, in among a grove of balsam poplars, I come up under the chevroned bark of an aspen. The black creases in the trunk all point skywards, like go-faster stripes for the eager climber; these are the points at which branches have been dropped by the tree, the 'eyelet' scars marking their former attachment.

I limber up on thin branches, climbing until the crown splits and the last arms of the aspen spray the sky. All around me pale-green leaves flutter in constant motion, the source of the aspen's 'quaking' nickname, rustling in the slightest breeze.

From high in the tree's rigging the whole expanse is laid out in miniature. Seagulls swoop in among scattered foot-ballers to pilfer half-time snacks and stray oranges. On the perimeter a thin band of mixed woodland is all that separates the marshes from the tower blocks beyond, a fragile dam holding back the tide of future development.

The Fallen Oak, Hampstead Heath
Quercus robur/English oak

A stone's throw from the north side of Parliament Hill stands a grove of oaks. In their midst is a tree felled in a bygone storm but saved from certain death by its crown; two prongs support it in a new horizontal life, the root base frozen half in, half out of the ground.

Climbing from this tangle of exposed anchors, I see that the oak is a well-travelled tree, its bark smooth and shiny with passage, like the feet of marble saints touched daily by the devout. The fissures on the bottom half of the trunk are completely flattened by this train of pilgrims.

I abandon my shoes and inch up on all fours. A copper-hued stub of a branch projects out to steady the climber, and a few more feet of crouched ascent gains the fork.

A choice of two paths presents itself. The angle at which the oak has come to rest creates twin arches, both ten feet off the ground. Following the left path, the climber embarks on a bridge crossing. Balancing on this oak high wire, I'm disorientated by the perspective; for a moment the branch could

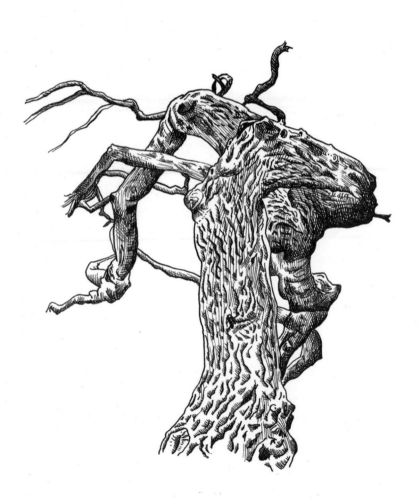

be lying flat on the soil and there is no sense of depth. Then a jogger whistles by beneath and I am floating over a mountain pass, the heath a distant valley floor.

On the far side of the bridge is a strange feature. A branch of the oak has grown back on itself, creating an enormous wooden jug handle. Sitting above this, I can dangle my feet through the hole and watch the path below me. Away to the north a stand of ragged Scots pines is a reminder of the native woodland that once flourished on the heath.

The tree's leaves nestle like shrubs on the ground, an inversion of their natural state. I imagine the oak suddenly righting itself, like tree felling played backwards, and being whisked forty feet or more into the air. In spite of the lack of cover up on the arches, few heath walkers glance up at my high seat. I return across the bridge, focusing on my hairy toes, then descend the tree by the second of the two paths. After a small distance this branch drops steeply away and I find myself sliding down, as if riding the banister of a grand staircase. With my face so close to the wood I discover a bark-coloured beetle with perfect grey-green camouflage. It scuttles away down the tree's underside as rain starts to spot the heath.

The Dule Tree, Wanstead Flats

Castanea sativa/Sweet chestnut

Walking out onto the Flats, I stop by an obelisk-shaped fountain dedicated to Joseph Fry: Quaker, banker and tea dealer. The marble is in a sorry state, a wet sock hanging over the lip and black spray paint covering the broken tap with the words 'Water please'.

I wade through long grass towards a small copse, one of several outliers of Epping Forest rooted on the common. The sun seems to have come to rest in Wanstead and the trees are illuminated like candle wicks, gold autumn leaves surrounding dark stems.

A dead stump arches out over the grass on the edge of the woodland, its underbelly white and bored with strange holes, the workings of rainwater or insect larvae. Climbing onto the topside, I walk up a deep channel of rotten wood filled with the dead leaves of neighbouring oaks. When I peel back a last shred of bark the stump reveals itself to be the remnants of a sweet chestnut. Spiders' eggs lie clustered in long seams that thread the grain.

This could be a dule tree, a 'tree of lament'. There is a long and ignoble history of using trees for improvised execution, and the jaunty angle of this branch would have made the perfect hangman's gallows. I perch tentatively on the apex; the deadwood feels solid under my weight, but for how much longer will it hold sway on the Flats?

As I journey on I see the spread arms of an English oak rise in the south-east corner of the next copse, its low crown

Jack Cooke

within easy reach. A hawthorn grows out of a cleft in the roots and its red berries match the mushrooms in the leaf litter – a warning flash of fly agaric. I hoist myself onto a stub at hip height before reaching to grasp a barrel branch overhead. The oak's crown is a fine specimen for lateral climbing and I traverse to its outer limits, patrolling the branches like a guard on a battlement.

Nearby a squirrel evades the stones of three children circling a beech by climbing out of their range. I follow suit, ascending to the highest branch in the hope of catching a London sunset.

Secret Gardens

We come at last to the forbidden Eden of tree-climbing, those cordoned-off segments of the city that blossom behind high walls and iron fence posts. Glimpsed through keyholes or the gaps in wooden slats, these private jungles grow in on themselves, occasionally thrusting a high arm out over the street.

When I pore over maps of London, four-walled sanctuaries appear like buried treasure in the folds of the city. Skirting their perimeters on foot, I listen for the sounds of what lies within, the breeze through a flower border or the thicket of a holly. Time is measured differently in these gardens and they can be anything our imagination desires, receptacles for childhood dreams. The draught escaping from under a door or through the bars of an ivy-wrapped gate is a blast of icy air, as if either might swing open onto rolling moorland or high hills. Passing a door with a rusted lock, long creepers climb cracked walls, like those guarding the rose garden where Lilias Craven fell from the branch of a tree in *The Secret Garden*. Anything could lie beyond – a land of never-ending summer or an empty lawn.

There is no greater temptation for the climber than these tantalising kingdoms, hanging over our heads like the fruit that ever eluded Tantalus himself. They remain behind bolt and key, and the only access to these secret realms is money, trespass or friends in high places.

If you part with a few coins, some of the greatest plantations in the city are open to you, gardens cultivated for hundreds of years with trees from every corner of the world. The nurseries of Kew and Chelsea are utopian spaces where the trees have taken firm hold, and their root world runs deep. These are places of learning not accustomed to seeing primates return to the canopy, so tread lightly across their sacred branches.

More enticing still are those cloistered squares sequestered in west London, the communal private gardens of Notting Hill, Kensington, Knightsbridge and Fulham, and few climbers can pass these riots of greenery without struggling against the urge to break and enter. When the leaves of overhanging branches brush against the world below, the power to resist ebbs away and we find ourselves ascending over the borderland between public and private. At first the climber trespasses in air space alone but, before long, the lure of other crowns draws them further in.

These are the gardens that inspired H. G. Wells to write his timeless ode to escapism, 'The Door in the Wall', a short story first published in 1911. Its protagonist, Lionel Williams, relates the tale of a secret garden he found as a child behind a long white wall with a green door, somewhere on the back roads of West Kensington. Stepping through, the boy discovers a magical interior, its long avenues of trees roamed by velvet panthers and fair-haired girls, and a flood of happiness overtakes him:

> *There was something in the very air of it that*
> *exhilarated, that gave one a sense of lightness and good*
> *happening and well being; there was something in the*
> *sight of it that made all its colour clean and perfect and*
> *subtly luminous … it was just like coming home.*

The space described in the secret garden is comparable to the space in the trees, a realm far removed from the hard realities of the city. Over the years, Williams stumbles on the green door time and again, but life always intervenes between him and his desire to return. He is a man 'haunted by something – that rather takes the light out of things, that fills me with longings …' and he fears the garden has been closed to him for ever. Williams struggles to maintain his public persona, the thought of that other world seeping into his every waking moment. Finally, driven to distraction, one dark night he steps through a door in the hoarding of a construction site, falling to his death in a deep excavation shaft beneath a railway. The story is a compelling parallel for the battle the tree climber wages between rational restraint and the lure of the imagination.

There is one further garden with fortified walls that I have long desired to explore: the forty-two acres of Buckingham Palace. The perimeter's high brick ramparts are topped with revolving spikes, barbed wire and a fleet of video cameras, and the trees beyond are giants undisturbed for centuries. I wrote to the Queen, asking to climb in her walled garden, and received a prompt reply declining my request but wishing me luck on my tree-top travels. Perhaps royals past have broken from numbing routine to escape up trees planted by their forebears, and maybe Elizabeth herself might once have been found perched in a pine, surveying the kingdom from a different throne.

A weekend in the calendar year for all explorers to cherish falls in June. 'Open Garden Squares Weekend' swings wide the gates to some of London's most exclusive addresses. Jealously guarded avenues and orchards are unbolted for a few short hours and open to all comers. Seize this moment to roam in the elevated greenery of these secret tree tops.

The Bowsprit, Rosmead Garden
Prunus avium/Wild cherry

If on a winter's night a traveller should pass by the silent gardens of Ladbroke Grove, they might be forgiven for hopping a fence …

I climb into Rosmead Garden over a different gate to the one Hugh Grant struggled up in *Notting Hill*, pleased that I manage it with a single attempt. Once inside, the last light of a December afternoon shines on a narrow green corridor, overhung with the bare fingers of horse chestnuts and the dead heads of willows.

The garden's by-laws, on a blackboard by the entrance, advise that 'Bows, arrows and catapults' are all strictly prohibited, but I have come unarmed. I tread cautiously across the lawn, searching for the outline of a climbing tree against the tall white façades of the terraced houses, pausing under each dark crown. Passing the frozen bars of a climbing frame, I hang for a moment, ears alert for the sound of others. But the garden remains hushed.

I settle for a cherry tree near the east end, a long arm jutting out of its bole like a spar from the foredeck of a ship. Climbing out along this, I feel the familiar ridges found in cherry bark; they are sharp against my hands and I pause to blow on cold knuckles. Further up, the branch has been pruned and a near-vertical shoot erupts from its tip, a scatter of branches stark against the sky. I think of Oscar Wilde's 'Selfish Giant' and the garden locked in winter, waiting for the children to climb back into its trees before blossoming again.

The sound of voices at the far end of Rosmead disturbs my reverie and, quickly, I drop from my perch and hide behind the wooden stakes of a Wendy house, grateful for the darkness now descending. Two, maybe three, figures pass by and leave through the gate, American accents lingering behind them.

Before making my escape I pause on a bench. Under the dim light of my torch ornate ironwork depicts swans gliding between wreathes of roses. The seat is dedicated to one Stefan Pinter, 'Fireworks maestro of Rosmead Garden for 21 explosive years'.

The Holy Holm, Lambeth Palace Gardens
Quercus ilex/Holm oak

The oldest cultivated garden in London is overshadowed by St Thomas' Hospital and bounded by Waterloo's rails. The sound of the city's drills, traffic and tourists seeps over the high brick walls, but the archbishop's rolling lawns remain a rare sanctuary.

A small door in the palace courtyard leads into the garden – ten acres of flowering borders and mature trees. I amble inside accompanied by a tide of tea-drinking nonagenarians, flocking through gates that open for just one day each month.

Beyond the stone terrace and the rose beds fronting the palace, a great spray of leaves erupts over the lawn. I quicken my pace at the sight of this evergreen crown, the marker of a long-rooted holm oak. Revealed in its entirety the tree does not disappoint, and its great reach casts a circular spell of shade across the garden. The crown bows towards the palace, supplicating itself to the ecclesiastical order.

In front of the trunk an old stem has been carved into a holy seat, with a conical back like a bishop's mitre and a cross etched into the wood. This rustic throne suggests some ancient rite, but enquiries with palace custodians reveal it to be the whim of the head gardener, clearly a wizard with a chainsaw.

I stand under the tree, its four thick fingers splaying upwards from the bole like a hand begging heaven for change. There are two obvious routes in: a running jump up the sloping side, or placing a hand in the crook of an elbow and balancing feet in the bark's crevices. Once well nested in the bole, the path to the best perch lies up the west-pointing arm directly above the bishop's wooden throne. I crawl up the first section before using a parallel branch overhead to steady my progress out along the limb, crab-walking to the tip. I wonder if the children of archbishops past or present have made this same aerial pilgrimage.

On one side the russet cone of a copper beech can be seen, another tree worth climbing, with a challenging ascent but a sturdy tangle of limbs at the summit. Close by, a black walnut planted by Queen Mary guards ground it has shadowed for over four hundred years. A small stone rotunda stands on a mound to the east of the tree. Beyond, the brick of a Victorian water tower soars above the garden walls.

The Widow's Veil, Chelsea Physic Garden
Fagus sylvatica 'Pendula'/*Weeping beech*

The entrance to this venerable old garden will give you small change from a tenner – ten pence, to be exact – but the treasures within are worth the price. Long a conduit for the passage of plants into Britain, the garden has many records to its name, including the first seeding cedar of Lebanon in 1732.

Although some unusual trees grow here – a fine cork oak and an olive – my favourite area in the garden is filled with herbs; name a disease and here lies a remedy, all laid out in meticulously ordered beds. The scents of medicinal plants from every corner of the globe pervade the garden's pathways.

Walking south, I pass a paper birch planted by Margaret Thatcher in 1988. It's tempting to shimmy up the bare trunk and wrestle with Maggie's crown, but the tree is a thin mast. A little further on, the fronds of a weeping beech envelop the south-east corner of the garden. I stoop to pass under the tree's shadow on the path, leaves brushing my back like a bead curtain. The beech is rooted next to the garden's study centre, and three upturned bottoms line the approach, the time-honoured pose of the horticulturalist.

Nearby an old man is watering a row of pot plants. He turns to smile at me and absentmindedly hoses a group of American tourists. Amid the ensuing confusion and apologies I step onto a log pile stacked against the tree and feel above me in the bole for a handhold.

The beech is like a mass of bunched muscle and its shoulders mimic those of the weary gardener. Once aloft I flat-palm my way up the southern arm, which thrusts out towards the boundary wall. The bole of the tree can reach immense proportions, growing secondary stems where the branch tips touch the ground.

A thick curtain of leaves hangs across the branch and the drone of Embankment traffic filters through from the far side. I stick my head through the drapery and find myself suddenly back in the city, a clogged highway below me and exhaust fumes all around. Pulling back, I am enclosed once more by the canopy and the peace of the walled garden. I play a game of peek-a-boo, ducking in and out, and try to catch the eye of a truck driver queuing alongside. Nothing will tempt his gaze away from the road, so I retreat into my lair and climb down.

The Prince of Persia, Kew Gardens
Quercus castaneifolia/Chestnut-leaved oak

Passing through Kew Gardens' imposing Victoria Gate, the questing climber experiences a rush of euphoria, for here lies an incomparable suburban Eden. Stretching in all directions, the high crowns of numberless trees reach for the heavens, and leaves of every shade compete for attention.

I leave my shoes in a border by the gate and set off barefoot across open lawns. Aside from a painful encounter with the spiked husk of a horse chestnut, the going is easy, and I walk on rolls of green velvet.

Climbing trees in Kew Gardens should be picked with care. I am intruding on an important planting site with many singular specimens, some of which deserve the distance accorded to paintings in galleries. Trees bounded by ropes must be given a wide berth, and any ascent where the climber is likely to cause damage avoided.

One giant whose polished lower limbs have seen the passage of many feet is the chestnut-leaved oak close by the Orangery. Although not the gardens' oldest or tallest example of the species, the tree has a majestic spread, branches beginning just above the ground and fanning into a broad crown. The oak is called 'chestnut-leaved' because its foliage resembles that of the sweet chestnut. Elliptic and serrated along their edges, they turn a deep bronze in autumn.

Quercus castaneifolia has strong limbs; the great storm of 1987 uprooted neighbouring trees but did not fell a single branch from this oak. I become completely absorbed in an endless procession around the lower reaches of the trunk, swinging under and over branches and lying flat on the wider beams. There are countless perches to choose from, and massive roots ripple through the woodchip floor below. The tree is far from its native soil in Iran but seems to be thriving under the care of Kew's gardeners.

An hour passes before I disentangle myself from the branches and walk out from under the tree's shadow. Looking back at the full spread of its crown, Kew Palace, the sometime home of King George III, looks dwarfed in the background, a red doll's house behind the oak stronghold.

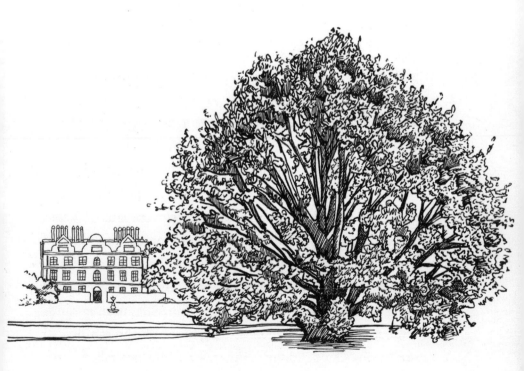

The Lost Dragon, Kew Gardens

Cedrus atlantica var. *glauca/Blue Atlas cedar*

The Cedar Vista is the longest single avenue in Kew Gardens and equal in majesty to the sweep of Whitehall or the grand march of The Mall. Looking along the length of its evergreen corridor, the stacked tiers of century-old cedars create a guarded space, a defence against the world outside.

I take a brief detour to the nearby 'Treetop Walkway', Kew's 2008 all-steel construction that allows visitors to climb into the canopy on metal rungs or take a lift. It's tempting to scale one of the old oaks or sweet chestnuts that rise to the level of the platform but their trunks offer no obvious paths to the top. What will happen when these trees reach the end of their life cycle and the walkway stands alone, bereft of purpose?

Back among the cedars I climb into a 'blue' Atlas, a variety planted for the powdery hue of its needles. The low arms of this specimen border the east end of the avenue, close by the garden's iconic pagoda.

Built in 1762, the pagoda rises ten storeys and one hundred and sixty-odd feet. Climbing in long loops around the cedar's trunk, I reach a branch level with the third of these floors and guess the tree to be sixty feet high. Framed between the cedar's fronds, the tower's sloping roofs look bleached and weather-worn. I am climbing on the eve of the building's restoration, a two-year programme to return the pagoda to its former majesty. Highlights include the promised return of

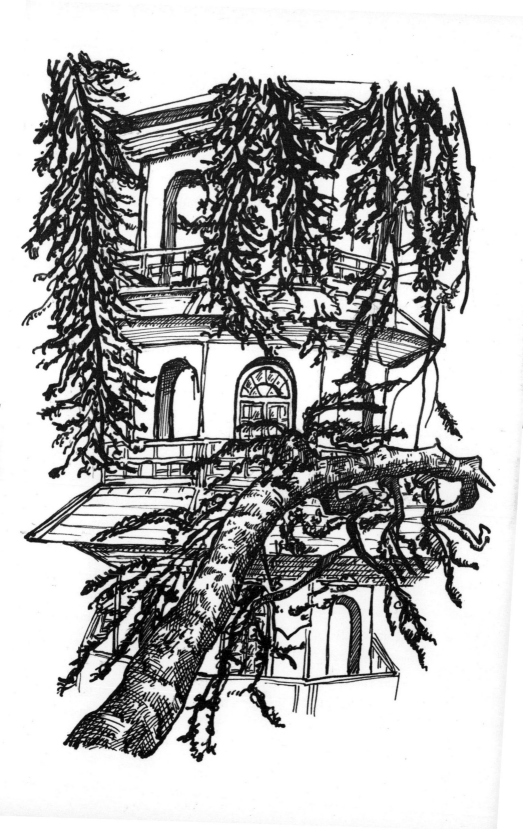

the dragons, eighty gilded monsters that last adorned the folly in the 1770s.

Looking down between my feet, I see the cedar's base is ringed with memorial benches. Scattered all over the four corners of Kew, many of these bear the same simple epithet: to men and women 'who loved these gardens'. It is a testament to Kew's riches that so many are commemorated in this way.

The Peacock Roost, The Hurlingham Club
Populus nigra 'Italica'/*Lombardy poplar*

I arrive, dressed in mandatory white, at the polished gates of the Hurlingham Club early on a Monday morning with the pretence of playing tennis.

Once inside I strike off along the Thames boundary, eyes peeled for a good climbing tree hiding in riverside obscurity. An old London plane with a heavy arm resting on the ground offers a low perch, but the trees nearby seem to be as immaculately trimmed as the club's grass tennis courts and croquet lawns.

Reaching the east end of the grounds, I cross the circle of a cricket field. On the far side is a striped blue and white marquee filled with empty pint glasses, the relics of a weekend's spectating.

Hard by the tent is the thin column of a Lombardy poplar. I reach up for a branch on the far side of the tree beneath a brick wall that separates the club from Broomhouse Lane.

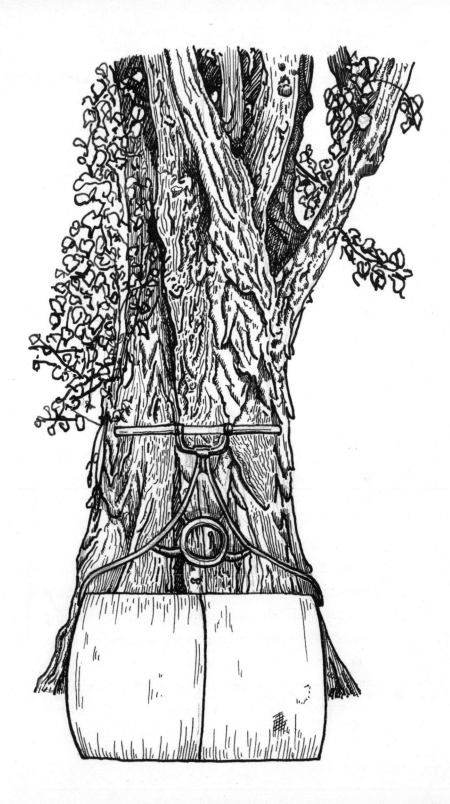

An old lawn roller rests against the trunk and I use its mighty barrel as a foothold. Above, the poplar's creviced bark provides enough purchase to struggle into its dense interior.

Lombardy poplars are awkward trees to climb. The branches are fastigiate, almost vertically aligned to the stem, forcing the climber to wedge their heels in the tight angles between. They are also brittle and prone to dropping their branches, but the high scaffolding of the 'Italian' poplar is irresistible. The trunk tapers and splits as I ascend but not before a bird's-eye view of the club appears, framed by diamond-shaped leaves. In the distance tennis players run along tramlines like white mice in a maze, while behind me construction traffic rumbles along the border of Hurlingham's private Eden.

In 1987 a Dutch artist called Marinus Boezem planted one hundred and seventy-four Lombardy poplars on a raised field in the Netherlands. His aim was to mimic the layout of Notre-Dame in Reims, creating a green cathedral out of this strangely uniform tree. Today, *De Groene Kathedraal*, complete with apse, aisles and ambulatory, has grown over one hundred feet high.

Climbing down, I almost fall out of the branches when serenaded by one of the club peacocks, its morning honk resounding like the blast of an air horn. Returning to the entrance, I pass beneath a redwood and alongside a colossal plane tree named after Captain Cook. Transformed by my adventure into a lime-green Grendel, I exit hurriedly past the suspicious eye of a security guard.

A Night Aloft

*The silence of the night when no breeze moved among
the watchful trees and everything seemed to be holding
its breath, or a night such as this, when all the winds of
heaven were up and out and every tree was pulling at its
anchor.*

Brendon Chase, B.B.

Entering Green Park at dusk through the funnel that leads
off St James's Place feels like stepping into another world.
Familiar pathways and avenues alter after dark and everything skews, objects looming impossibly close or shrinking
into the distance. London at night is virgin territory for me,

like the walled yard in *Tom's Midnight Garden* that transforms on the stroke of twelve into a magical escape. The touchstones of the day are indecipherable in a world drained of colour.

I have come to the park tonight to climb one last tree. With me is Isam, an old friend and conspirator, and between us we carry some unusual implements. We walk close together in the gloaming, the whole city seeming to cool and contract with the onset of night. Distances resolve slowly in the twilight, as if the ground we step on does not exist until the moment of our passing.

An unclimbable tower has lured me here, a beech whose lowest branches sail agonisingly out of reach fifteen feet above the lawn. It rises near the park's northern boundary, hard by the highway of Piccadilly, and the upper branches form a ladder disappearing into an invisible tree top, a crow's nest holding sway over central London. The beech has become an obsession ever since an idea took root in my head: to spend a night sleeping in a tree.

On a breathless summer night, lying awake in my flat with the window open, I listened to the single ash left on Ashfield Street, trying to catch any trace of a breeze in its branches. The greasy advance of hot tyres and the bass notes of car stereos seeped into my room and the heat of the day festered. Outside, night cooled the pavements and alleyways. I had fitful dreams of time spent in the trees, of swaying branches and broad sunshades made from leaves. Waking, stifled by the stale air of the bedroom, I ran through all those I had climbed over the preceding months. Their elevated bowers seemed the perfect retreat from the claustrophobia of my room. Which of them would I not swap for my own sprung mattress?

A host of green escapes suggested themselves: the cedar in Greenwich Park with its perfect cocoon in the solitude of fenced acres, the city no more than a glimmer on the skyline; the pine deep in Brompton Cemetery, silent as the dead lying beneath it; the private crown of the beech in Fulham Palace Gardens; the lonely plane tree on Tooting Common. These and others appealed, for the kind geometry of their branches or for their seclusion, far from sirens, street lights and pub crawls.

The next morning I reviewed the candidates. For all the temptation of these reclusive roosts my choices were symptomatic of a desire to escape London entirely, and I might as well have caught a train to the New Forest and roped myself to the crown of an old oak. I could spend a night watching the moon rise over a canopy haunted by owls, listening to badgers root around on the forest floor.

And yet there was another kind of life I wanted to observe, deep in the city itself: the nocturnal wandering of my fellow city dwellers. I needed a watchtower not a nest, a way of spying on London through the small hours and charting the night cycle of the city.

The beech is perfect for my purpose, having borne silent witness to a century of comings and goings. Many of London's green retreats close their gates at dusk, but Green

Park remains open twenty-four hours and anyone can traverse its lanes day or night. The park is at the city's core, sandwiched between main roads and busy thoroughfares, its inner acres lying undisturbed. It is at once the centre and antithesis of the urban, haunted by the sound and light of passing traffic but dark and shadowed within.

The tree requires tools for a nocturnal climb and a dawn descent. We make our way west along the darkening avenues, an odd couple, the Arab with the ladder and the Saxon with a rope. Gas lamps flicker into life, casting our suspect silhouettes across the park's open spaces. The temperature is cooler than on the street and the wind hums through the canopies high above us. Approaching the beech, the last light is sucked from the park's fringe. A cyclist passes us in the gloom, her blinking lights like the pyrotechnic core of a deep sea fish. She vanishes over a rise with a farewell flash of red and we step under the thrall of the tree's leaves where night has already fallen.

With care, Isam erects the ladder against the pillar of the beech, glancing around us for fear of watchmen. We are well concealed, the spreading foliage of the tree sweeps to within a metre of the ground and only our legs remain visible to the outside world. He motions and I step up onto the first rung. Hand over hand the darkness deepens and instead of climbing I feel like I descend into lightless waters. As I reach the last tread, the ladder's feet slip on the uneven ground around the roots. The world shifts sideways and I clasp the trunk, my feet sliding out from under me. In that dreadful, suspended second I see myself lying sprawled amongst the tree's unforgiving feet, a foolish man who tried to climb blind. Thankfully the scaffold is steadied, and a moment later I have left London behind, trusting my hands and feet to the thick arms of the beech.

The steps drop away in the dark and, instinctively, I begin climbing higher, feeling my way from branch to branch as my eyes adjust to the gloom within. Remembering my friend, I look back beneath my legs. Far below I can just make out the glimmer of the retracting ladder, but already Isam seems impossibly distant. 'Good night' drifts up from the shades of the park and he is gone. The beech is now my sole companion for the hours of darkness.

Green Park is a domain ruled by trees. Few flowers grow in their shade and no borders burst with bright colour. It is a cathedral space after dark, wooden columns rising into the soft pink ceiling of the city sky at night. Silhouetted branches soar overhead like the forked ribs of medieval vaults, and voices from behind trees sound like Gregorian chant.

Adrenalin helps me through the first twenty feet of the climb. The branches are barely visible and my route, plotted from the ground in daylight, is a lost map to me now. A poem by David Wagoner seeps into my mind:

The only guides are the heart in my mouth,
My body's guesswork,
And sticks crackling under my feet as if in a dark fire.

I climb to a ring of thick limbs growing around the trunk's circumference and grab hold of a branch like a jug handle on the south side of the tree. Clinging to this reassuring anchor, I let my eyes adjust to the darkness. I have come further than I think, and below me is a false floor; what I had imagined to be the ground is a new plantation of trees growing alongside the beech, their tops fanning out beneath.

I begin again, deciding to push as far as I dare before settling on a perch for the night. The drop is less real now and I climb disembodied, my immediate hand- and footholds the only tangible objects in a world of grey hues. The ascent seems never-ending, and I imagine climbing on for mile after mile, like Jack on his beanstalk. But then, at long last, I come to a nest of branches, a platform high on the flank of the tree with a window on to the city.

Gas lamps pool dim circles of light far below, like the sun-bleached slides of an old carousel, stark against the park's black-velvet vegetation. I tie myself to a branch with a sling brought for the purpose – it's a fine thing to be unencumbered in the tree tops, but no monkey's tail will save me should I fall asleep during my vigil. Once secured I am filled with new confidence and walk far out on the branch, my hands steadied on a beam above. This is all that separates me from the sky, two hard black lines in an amphitheatre of pure air. Standing there, forty feet or more above the park, I am suspended outside time. I look down on the city's lights, half-lit towers on the horizon and halogen-flooded walkways along Piccadilly. The park lawn is a jigsaw of shadow.

The beech fills me with a sense of security and becomes a great confidant in the night. When all around is cold space and all below unseen, the bark is a rough but reassuring presence. Once again I think of my fictional hero from *The Baron in the Trees*, the tree-dwelling Cosimo, 'He who spent his nights listening to the sap germinating from cells, the circles marking the years inside the trunks, the mould enlarging its patches quivering under the north wind.' Returning to my high seat, I slump with my back against the trunk and my legs straddling a branch like a saddle.

Green Park's history is laced with gunpowder, a legacy of fireworks and blood feuds settled with duels. It was not always a space so devoid of buildings, and great temples once adorned its interior. The Temple of Peace and the Temple of Concord stood proud in its midst, colonnades of marble and stone with grand terraces, but both were doomed by fire. The first was used to store ten thousand fireworks for a celebration in 1749. A stray rocket landed inside the temple and set the entire magazine alight, creating a giant fireball that burnt the edifice – and several bystanders – to cinders. No lesson was learnt, and sixty-eight years later the same fate befell the Temple of Concord during celebrations for the Prince Regent's gala. From the vantage of the beech I look out across the lawn and see these great blazes of the distant past, cyclones of flame tearing through the centre of the park. Horses scream in the heat and crowds scatter from lone figures set on fire, reeling like mad puppets amid the pandemonium.

An ambulance passing down Piccadilly tears me back into the present; its lights make a thousand leaves sparkle blue.

* * *

The beech is a two-faced tree, one side exposed to the road and the other turned towards the sanctuary of the park. I wonder if a great migration takes place after sundown, nocturnal denizens shunning the street's reflected light and seeking dark crevices to the south. As if on cue, two earwigs drop into my hair, reaffirming that I am not the sole occupant. My clothes are a poor second skin and some other insect, unaccustomed to cotton, is charting an invisible passage up the inside of my arm.

The crown of the beech forms a black tent overhead and the leaves are a fine choice of canvas. Staring through their still hordes, I feel part of an intricate design, as if caught up in the tree's tapestry and bound to remain there for an eternity. My eyes follow the foliage down through the branches and into the impenetrable understorey. The River Tyburn runs directly beneath the park soil; in medieval times it was little more than a swamp, serving as a burial ground for lepers from the Hospital of St James the Less. Into this soggy grave their bodies were sunk by the hundred. My thoughts drift down to the root world of the beech and I shudder to think what lies long entangled beneath.

The hours catch up with me and I try to sleep with my face turned down between two branches, the tree falling away like an endless staircase. Although the view does not frighten me, freed as it is from any sense of perspective, every time I start to drift my body jerks awake, fighting for balance. How many nights of hanging here would it take before my bones adapt to a nest in the tree top? The beech wood has cooled beneath me, sapping my body heat, and before long I'm shivering.

Between this intermittent dozing I wonder if anyone has passed on the path close by the beech, confused by human snores emanating from high overhead. There is a legend that tells of a death – or doom – tree, growing somewhere in Green Park, under whose branches the fated fall asleep, never to wake again. Perhaps I will foster a new legend, of a nasal ghost dwelling in the canopy of the park.

I banish sleep with the help of a Kendal mint cake and shed my diurnal body for a new alter ego: a sentry watching the night. To the north, across Piccadilly's four lanes of traffic, the balconies of the Park Lane Hotel are illuminated. I stare at the dead-eyed glaze of the hotel's windows and wonder if anyone is awake and looking out at the park. Do they long to sail on imaginary wings from their high window and over the soft verge of the lawn? Or are they happy watching re-runs and emptying the mini-fridge? My own perch is level with the fourth floor of the building, where a suite starts at £500 a night. I've lost all feeling in my legs but take pride in my penthouse.

While opening a bag of mixed nuts from the larder in my rucksack, I see a figure move into the circle of light under a gas lamp, like a scene from an old film noir. Something falls from their coat and the sound of glass breaking echoes out across the park, loud as a revolver's report. They mutter something unintelligible then walk quickly away, shoulders hunched.

When the echo fades I become aware of all the other small sounds of the park slowly creeping back into my consciousness: the fidgeting of pigeons in the tree top, the creak of a branch and, somewhere, the sound of running water. Different spheres of sound fan out from the beech and my inner ear tunes into these, like the loose wheel of a radio. Near at hand the immediate life of the tree is filled with movements beneath the canopy, twigs snapping and leaves rustling. Further afield are the sounds of the park, footsteps on pathways and litter blown across open spaces. Beyond, the bass hum of the wider city prevails, the sigh of bus exhausts and the voices of distant crowds. By starting small and moving outwards I feel I can project my hearing half a mile or more, listening in to encounters on street corners and mapping the architecture of the city with my ears alone.

Wrapped around the tree I get the uncanny feeling that the branches are human limbs, the wooden knuckles under my hands and thighs the joints of another body. The beech is unassailable, but sinister figures begin to take shape in the boughs beneath me. Spider-like forms climb up to snatch at my dangling legs and hairy talons thread the branches overhead. Perhaps this is an ancient apprehension, the collective memory of a time when our ancestors were stalked in this way, or it might just be the fear of monsters under the bed transposed to a tree.

Such horrible images are doubly unsettling in the dark as my eyes cannot focus straight ahead. Colour-perceiving cones are concentrated in the centre of our retinas and rendered useless at night. Only the rod cells work, the grey receptors clustered around the perimeter. We become like rabbits, with eyes set on either side of our skulls, haunted by objects at the edges of our peripheral vision.

My nightmares fade with the imperceptible brightening of the eastern horizon, a deep indigo emerging from the black veil over Westminster. I feel like an astronaut or submarine pilot, returning by blue degrees to the surface of the world.

Just before dawn I move higher until I gain a perch like the prow of a ship. Facing due east, the branch yaws in a stiff breeze and London seems to part before the bow wave of the beech, which breaks free from its roots and sails out across the city. As the tree sways beneath me and the light strengthens I'm aware for the first time in hours of the great drop under my feet. With what ease might I fall, like a sailor from his masthead into a rolling sea of green.

A wood pigeon calls from a neighbouring tree but sounds unsure of himself, his cries soon lost in the first rush of morning traffic along Piccadilly. Stumbling unseen through the park below, a drunk starts his own dawn chorus, a burst of short hallelujahs that acts like a call to arms; suddenly the park is alive with birdsong. The lone hoot of a tawny owl is the last voice of the night before a host of crows unlock the morning with loud caws. The insect life of the park is hard on their shoulders – a large bee cartwheels in front of me but is soon lost to the sky.

As morning arrives a wonderful smell rises up the tree from below. I soon recognise the familiar aroma of coffee, drifting downwind from the styrofoam cup of a passing commuter, and the smell provokes an animal hunger in me.

Stiff in every limb, I cautiously thread my way back down. The gaps between branches widen and the beech feels like a very different tree to the one I climbed at night. After much indecision I reach the final branch before the drop-off. The light is growing with every passing minute, and I'm keen to be down and away before the park wardens begin their morning rounds. Beneath me the emptiness is imposing and I hope to hell I've bought sufficient rope. Sitting astride the branch and uncoiling the line from my rucksack, I hold on to it with white knuckles, knowing it is my only way down. Inch by inch I play out the rope and draw the two strands on either side together. With relief I see the frayed ends kiss the ground. I've no patience for knots and trust that my carabiner will ensure a safe descent. Before heaving myself off the edge I take a final look back up through the branches at my former roost. The whole interior of the tree is suffused with light and somewhere far above I have left an unmade bed.

I am no elegant abseiler and bounce down the side of the trunk, burning my hands with the rope. Above me the white cord vanishes over the topside of the branch, like the trail Theseus once laid in the labyrinth. I pull on the rope, it falls back to earth, and the beech stands impregnable once more.

Back on the ground someone has left a pair of wet boxers buried in the tree roots, and a collection of graffiti scars the base of the trunk. Angela, or her admirer, has carved her name boldly across the whole girth, and next to this is a hashtag with the numerals five two six. The contrast of a Twitter call sign with the permanence of the tree is a hard wrench back into the modern world.

I coil the rope in a daze, my feet in the park but my mind elsewhere, roaming the silver skyways of the beech. A morning begun in the canopy is a different prospect to one approached through bed rest. My body aches from root to crown and walking once-familiar streets I feel a race apart. Buses and taxis pass me by, my reality still in the trees; a window to an older world has opened for me and a memory of the primeval lingers, the stain of mould on my fingers, the scent of sap in my clothes.

The Sprouting City

Now it was a whole different world, made up of
narrow curved bridges in the emptiness, of knots
or peel or scores roughening the trunks, of lights
varying their green according to the veils of thicker
or scarcer leaves.

The Baron in the Trees, Italo Calvino

If we climb a tree and spend five minutes among its branches, we can barely claim to know it. The examples in this book reward return visits, so that we see them in different seasons and at different times of day. The longer we spend in any given tree, the more we adjust to its rhythms. In time we come closer to the natural order, bird and beast willingly returning to the branches around us.

A strange sense of possession comes from climbing trees that few, if any, other people ever visit. Retracing our way along a favourite branch, we are the sole witness to its daily changes. Inhabiting an oak for an hour, we have travelled further than a few feet off the ground, crossing into territory that we alone charter. Our chosen trees become objects we cling to, personal landmarks in an urban environment that is often deeply alienating.

The trees in this book are fixed in my memory, whatever their future, but I am under no illusion that they will always welcome me back. If we open old records of the city's great trees, former praise now reads like sad eulogy; searching for their traces, too often I find ground filled in or built over. Pursuing their trail is like navigating London's buildings using a guide published before the Blitz.

Trees are never still. They grow and shrink, their appearance changing with the passing months and years. They may shed branches and remove themselves from the climber's eager grasp, or succumb to the dangers of living – age, disease and accident. They might be cut down by lightning or dug up by developers, but for every fallen branch another will sprout. If you journey to the foot of a tree in this book to find it no longer there, take heart; the arboreal metropolis that grows through and above the city will replenish itself, new trees inviting passers-by to step up into their arms. A silent growth permeates the city, and it continues without the aid of cranes or power tools.

Sometimes I daydream a different London where every man-made structure has been swept away. Sinkholes swallow pavements, earthquakes crack steel and glass. The map is laid bare; office blocks, tenements and stations cease to exist. In my fantasy, London's trees remain standing in this new desert. What would the city look like with its contours revealed, the river twisting through scattered groves and ringed by wooded hills?

After days spent holding carriage or escalator handrails, touching bark is bracing like a shock of cold water. No other surface compares to living wood and climbing brings a feeling of reversion, a step back from a wholly artificial environment. By scaling trees we unpick the city, bridging the divide between the life we lead and the life we led long ago.

There exists a halfway realm between the fixed fabric of our urban landscape and the constant movement of its inhabitants. Trees are stationary but alive, and being neither fully static nor animate gives them a powerful attraction. One moment they are lost in the background of the street, no different to a lamp post or a steel girder; the next they form a living roof over our heads. In this way trees act as mediators between the city dweller and the natural world, an ever-present reminder of what lies under the paved and tarmacked crust.

Tree climbing is a curious form of travel. Ascending, we cross the divide between two worlds and the people passing beneath us become as separate as fish in an aquarium. Discovering a trunk with a clear path to the crown is enticing as finding a ladder to the moon; this is the essence of climbing, a method of passing between two spheres – the humdrum everyday and the elevated.

Putting physical space between ourselves and our daily routines cannot be overvalued. Tree tops are spaces that renew our appreciation for small pleasures, and being aloft magnifies the commonplace: reading a book, talking to a friend or enjoying a cup of airborne coffee. Sitting on a branch provides a kind of momentary amnesia, an immersion in the natural world that allows us to forget street-level worries. The canopy is a place of quiet revelation, and when we sit alone in the greenwood, a new solitude is experienced – not the isolation of an indifferent city but the solace of clear thought. People move through the street looking through a wide-angle lens, hyperaware of peripherals but ignoring the trees growing in their midst. Crossing a road or making a phone call, we are too preoccupied to look up. By climbing trees we can apply a microscope to our surroundings, suddenly the smallest textures of bark and branch captivate our attention.

Writing this book has served to keen my senses. The trees have become destinations in themselves, living monuments as fundamental as any other landmark. Little by little, they have encroached on my image of the city and sown chaos in a cloistered life.

A city can be reduced to its parts and we can focus on what we wish to. By attuning yourself to the trees, you draw a new, personal map of your environment, predicated on networks of oak, ash and beech, rather than transport links or the opening hours of shops. My search for different trees has taken me to corners of London I would otherwise have passed by and to space I never knew existed. Stepping off a bus or out from the Underground, my first thought is to scan the street for its trees, learning to recognise crowns from afar and straying to catalogue new climbs.

Exploring in this way is the most tangible connection we have to our childhood. Trees provide the missing link to the awe of our early years, when our love of nature was unfettered. If we can awaken the impish child in all of us, we can learn to cast off simulated lives and get back to enjoying the living world around us. Like the truant hiding in a treehouse, we must train ourselves not to come down when civilisation calls.

Climbing trees becomes an obsession. Like the ivy that prises open a window, trees have taken over the order of my days. Commuting on overground trains, I dream of pulling alarms to stop by embankments where tall oaks grow. Staring longingly at tree tops, I walk into lamp posts and trip over kerbs. The shapes of trees begin to appear in everything; when I run my hand along a wooden banister my fingers seem to ply high branches; eyeing broccoli on a dinner plate, I long to shrink to the size of an ant and explore its glorious green boughs. No longer content to exist in a fixed world, I am forever searching for a way up.

There is no end to the canopy that threads the city, and the climber would need the lifespan of a sequoia to reach the final branch. Many grails still elude me: a green corner of

London where two climbable trees grow side by side, allowing passage from one into the next, or a high branch that overhangs a balcony. These and other daydreams distract from the task of living. Venture too often into the trees and you risk becoming the Green Man of legend, leaves sprouting from mouth and ears, forever bound to the vegetable world.

Living in the city, a vital part of us becomes sedated and our natural instincts are subdued. We take our urban environment for granted and ignore the organic empire that grows under and over it. The city becomes more crowded by the day but we must not allow our need for space to crowd out the trees themselves. The finest architecture is a wasteland without an interval of branches, and if we fail to accommodate the trees we are in danger of suffocating in a lung-less world. Our interactions with nature need not be confined to airbrushed adverts or watching mice running over rail lines – the canopy forms an aerial chain for wildlife to move across the city and the climber can follow in their wake.

Abandon the narrow cartography of your phone and try looking on the world from the vantage of a branch. You might be surprised at the vision that presents itself. Whether hanging over London, or high above a hedgerow in some distant field, thousands of green towers await your ascent. Climb often and climb widely, and you will gain a country all of your own, a secret garden in the sky.

Branching Out –
A Tree Climber's
Glossary

For those who wish to steep themselves in the word lore of the trees, a lifetime's study awaits. The terms below represent only the topsoil of a vast, diverging root system. Some are botanical, others purely fanciful – any number of descriptive words can be applied to the endless variety of climbing trees.

Apex
From the Latin, meaning a 'point, tip or summit'. In botany the apex refers to the ends of leaves, petals or branches. Venturing out towards the apex of a branch is a goal for bold climbers and a bit like walking the plank. Tread carefully.

Arboreal

Relating to or resembling a tree. Also 'living among the trees'. I like to think that an arboreal state of mind exists – a new consciousness that's acquired after a day spent among branches.

Bole

From the Old Norse word *bolr*, meaning 'tree trunk', or the Old English *bolla* for a 'pot, cup or bowl'. This is the branchless bottom of the trunk, and a living cliff to conquer.

Burr

A burr is a rounded projection growing from a tree. Usually the result of damage or stress, these bulbous growths chart a tree's physical history – a bit like human dental records. Burrs can provide much-needed purchase for the climber; some wrap around an entire trunk while others project like warts from the bark. Interestingly, burr wood is prized by furniture makers – when cut, its twisted grain reveals intricate patterns.

Cambium

Derived from the medieval Latin for 'change or exchange', this is the living layer of plant tissue between bark and wood, and a vital transport network for the tree. Nutrients pass up from the roots and food passes down from the leaves. When the cambium layer is exposed by man or beast, the tree withers. A circle of naked cambium around a trunk's circumference is known as 'ring barking' and results in the premature death of the tree (commonplace where young saplings are exposed to grazing animals).

Canker

Cankers are the result of fungal and bacterial infections, causing bark to split into deep fissures. These intricate scars look like open wounds in the wood. Often found on the top sides of branches, climbers sometimes discover cankers that remain invisible from the ground.

Canopy

The canopy is the tree's upper layer of leaves and a living roof over the climber's head. When a tree is in leaf, this green ceiling is the ultimate escape from the world at street level.

Catkin

From the obsolete Dutch *katteken*, meaning 'kitten'. Catkins are the flowering spikes that appear on many species prior to spring leaves, dangling like earrings from the ends of branches.

Conifer

Derived from the Latin *conus*, meaning 'cone-bearing'. Nearly all conifers are evergreen, retaining their leaves all the year round. An exception in this book is the swamp cypress, *Taxodium distichum* (see *The Royal Perch, St James's Park*).

Coppice

From the medieval Latin *colpus*, meaning 'a blow'. Trees that have been coppiced are cut back to the *bole*, reduced to a stump from which new branches sprout. This is a time-honoured technique, enabling foresters to harvest wood while prolonging the life of the tree through constant regeneration. Some trees have multiple stems sprouting from the ground, a likely consequence of past coppicing (see *The Tree of Knowledge, Richmond Park*).

Copse

A small stand or group of trees, often isolated (see *Gwain's Bane, Wormwood Scrubs* or *The Dule Tree, Wanstead Flats*).

Crook

From the Old Norse *krokr*, meaning 'hook', and referring to the join between branch and stem, a reassuring place for the climber to rest. For comfort and security, nothing compares to sitting in the crook of a tree with your back against the trunk.

Crown

The crown of a tree begins with the first branch and encompasses the entire structure, growing outwards from a central axis. Recognising the geometry of different crowns, the climber can identify tree species from a distance.

Deciduous

From the Latin verb *decidere*, meaning 'to fall down'. This category comprises all species that shed their leaves in autumn.

Dendrochronologist

If you've ever idly tried counting the growth rings on the exposed *heartwood* of a tree, you can call yourself a dendrochronologist. Pay special attention to the space between each circle; this tells you how much the tree grew in any given year, and a narrow ring is a sure sign of hard times.

Fastigiate

Having branches more or less parallel to the main stem, as typified by the Lombardy poplar, *Populus nigra* 'Italica'. Fastigiate trees make for painful ascents, forcing the climber to wedge a heel between branch and trunk.

Fork

Where a branch splits into two at the tip. A useful prop for climbing into a tree and, higher up, a double perch for friends exploring together.

Glaucous

From the Greek *glaukos*. In botany, 'covered with a bluish waxy or powdery bloom' (also the name of a sea god with a fish tail …). Typified by the dusty blue-green needles of the Atlas cedar variety, *Cedrus atlantica* var. *glauca* (see *The Lost Dragon, Kew Gardens*).

Granny Pine

A special appellation given to mature, multi-branched Scots pine, *Pinus sylvestris*, bent over by age or weather. 'Granny' specimens are noted for their chaotic, wayward branches (see *The Granny Pine, Paddington Old Cemetery*).

Heartwood

The dense inner part of a tree trunk. Often darker than *sapwood* and yielding a harder timber.

Hollow

From the Old English *holh*, meaning 'cave'. Used here to describe the cavities in trees that provide useful hand- and footholds for the climber.

Hybrid

Cross-breeding of different species to create new varieties and cultivars. This occurs naturally in some wild trees, but is also commonplace in cultivation to produce desired characteristics. Two examples in these pages are the London plane, *Platanus* × *acerifolia*, and the hybrid black poplar, *Populus* × *canadensis* (see *The Oasis, Blackheath*).

Knot

From the Old English *cnotta*, meaning 'an intertwining of ropes or cords'. A common blemish, knots are found on the stem, branches and roots of a tree. Knots come in many forms, from hard, lumpy protrusions to small holes in the bark. Also referred to as 'gnarls', hence 'a gnarled old tree'. Knots are the climber's consolation on branchless trunks, where nothing else offers a way up.

Native

A term reserved for those brave species that re-colonised Britain after the retreat of the ice sheet at the end of the last glacial period (see *Species* for fuller explanation).

Palmate

Leaves arranged like the fingers of a human hand, though not restricted to five digits. The horse chestnut, *Aesculus hippocastanum*, is a classic example.

Pinnate

A leaf with leaflets arranged in two ranks along a shared axis. Ashes, rowans and walnuts all conform to this pattern, creating verdant canopies for the climber.

Pollard

Possibly derived from the Low German *poll*, meaning 'head', this is the method of cutting off the top branches of a tree to encourage upward growth. Differs from *coppicing* in that the branches are usually cut eight or more feet above the ground.

Prune

Any technique for trimming a tree, including *pollarding*. Cutting away dead or overgrown branches or stems, not only to increase fruitfulness and growth but also to clear paths and roadways. In the city, overpruning is the council's prerogative and the climber's curse.

Resin

Sticky, water-insoluble and highly flammable, resin is a tree's defence system and exactly what you don't want glued to your hands. Commonly produced by cedars, firs and pines, the *conifer* climber is lucky to escape without a fine coating.

Sapwood

Soft, living layers of wood, formed between *heartwood* and bark and containing sap, the lifeblood of the tree. Also the basis of a curious, 19th-century insult – 'sap-skull' – used to deride a gullible person.

Sucker

A shoot springing from the surface root of a tree. When multiple, well-established suckers surround a parent tree, the climber has a private forest to play in.

Taper

Reducing in thickness towards one end. Used to describe the thinning of a branch or stem.

Tendril

A term usually applied to climbing plants such as vines, denoting a slender, thread-like appendage. In some mature trees with curling branches, the climber threads a maze of super-sized tendrils.

Tresses

From the Old French *tresce*, meaning 'a lock of hair'. Applied here to any tree with cascading foliage, such as white weeping willow, *Salix × sepulcralis*.

Tusking

A branch sloping steeply upward from the main stem, like the tusks of an elephant. Shallower angle than *fastigiate* limbs.

Whorl

Curling, swirling, spiralling or coiling – a wonderful word. In botany, a whorl refers to a radiating pattern of leaves or petals. It could just as well sum up the whole experience of climbing trees.

Understorey

The layer of vegetation beneath the main canopy of a forest or wood. Some tree species are well adapted to thriving in the shadow of others (see *Brothers in arms, Bishop's Park*).

Acknowledgements

First and foremost to my wife Jennifer, whose beautiful illustrations capture the joy of exploring bark and branch far better than words; my wonderful agent Claudia Young, for her enthusiasm from beginning to end; Jack Fogg, editor and mastermind, and Mark Bolland, copyeditor and naturalist – both who made this book infinitely better than it would otherwise have been; finally, Fergus Kinmonth, whose expertise helped identify the species of various trees climbed in woeful ignorance.

The Tree Climber's Guide

Field Notes

286

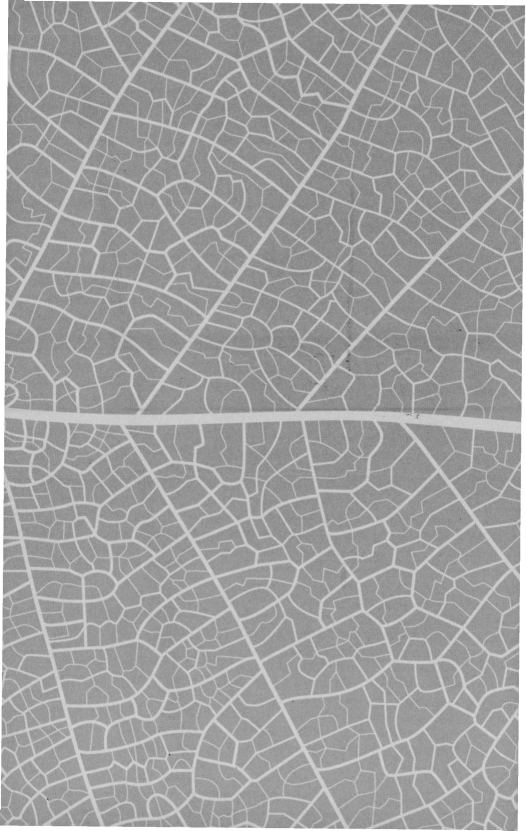